# Learning to Be You; It's an Inside Job

## *Recovery and Healing for the Loved Ones of the Substance-Addicted*

**Brenda Ehrler**

**Second Edition, Revised**

Just Be Publishing, Inc. ✕ Salt Lake City, Utah

# Learning to Be You; It's an Inside Job

*Recovery and Healing for the Loved Ones of the Substance Addicted*

**By Brenda Ehrler**


First Printing 1999
Second Printing 2000, revised

Published by:
**Just Be Publishing, Inc.**
P.O. Box 571176
Murray, UT 84157-1176
Printed in the United States of America
**Publishers Cataloging-in-Publication Data**
Ehrler, Brenda
Learning to be You; It's an Inside Job: Recovery and Healing for the Loved Ones of the Substance-Addicted / by Brenda Ehrler.
cm. p.
Included bibliographical references.
ISBN 0-9668219-2-0 (pbk.): $13.95
1. Substance abuse—Family relationships 2. Self-care 3. Self-actualization I. Title
158'.1 CIP 98-094072
ISBN 0-9668219-2-0

# TABLE OF CONTENTS

# ACKNOWLEDGMENT

I would like to thank my family for their trust in my abilities. I am especially thankful for my husband's support and acceptance of this book. There would be no story without his recovery and subsequent healing.

I would like to acknowledge my son, Sy Ehrler, who created the picture that appears on the cover. With his unique creative vision, he interpreted my description of what I wanted, and gave me more than I could have imagined.

Also, I would like to thank my daughter, Adryen, for her insightful suggestions. She gave me "thumbs-up" after reading the first chapters of the book. Her encouragement was both meaningful and timely.

**Edited by:**

Ben Mates

**Critiqued by:**

Rita Robinson,Writer's Digest Criticism Service

**Readers:**

Cynthia Jones, Linda Marquez, Joyce Luker and Betty Jo Bartlett

**Photograph of the Author:**

Dave Labrum, Master Photographer, C.P.P., Busath Photography, Salt Lake City, Utah

Thanks to the following, for their technical and administrative assistance:

Coilin Brown, Syncnet, Salt Lake City, Utah

Ramona Rudert, Executive Director of the Women's Business Center, Salt Lake Area Chamber of Commerce.

*This book is dedicated to our sweet kitten, Miracle. She left her physical body on February 26, 1999, but only after she had crept into the heart of each family member.*

*This revised edition is dedicated to Sebastian, our Miniature Schnauzer. He left his physical body to move on to his next phase of existence on October 26, 1999.*

# INTRODUCTION

*There are no accidents in life just a continuation of experiences building toward a grand finale. If you think this book is speaking to you, it is.*

I wrote this book for the friends and family members of drug and alcohol addicted individuals. I have experienced the pain associated with the addiction of a loved one. In 1980, I met and married my husband, who is a drug addict and alcoholic. He used drugs and alcohol until 1990 and has been clean and sober since. I will share how we moved into healing, not only the outer manifestation of the addiction but also the inner conditions that brought them about.

If you are a friend or family member of an alcoholic or drug addict, you might have a story similar to mine. You might have picked up this book hoping that you will find comfort within its pages. I believe you will find comfort, but not in the way you might expect. I'm not going to give you a list of situational do's and don'ts. Nor will I tell you that the discomfort you are experiencing will go away. I will give you ideas on how to change your perceptions, and thus change your life.

I ask for your non-judgement as you read this book. I will share many details about my own family's dysfunction as we struggled with the disease of addiction. I do so to help you to find further understanding with your own life experiences.

# Chapter 1

## The End and the Beginning

*I had been reading books about people who had had guns pointed at them, and I wondered why they just didn't take off, so that's what I did.*

The headline read "Wife's Car Shot, Husband Arrested." That is the end of our end, and the true beginning of our new beginning.

Joe is drunk when he picks me up from work. He drinks almost every other day. Therefore that day is typical for him, but something has changed in me. On the two-mile country ride home, I try to explain to Joe my belief that we have been unsuccessfully trying to change one another for the last nine and a half years.

"Joe, I'm tired of the way we are living. Maybe it would be better if we just split up. You can go your way, and drink all you want. I can go mine and stop the constant complaining."

Joe doesn't like my suggestion. He reacts in the same way he always does when confronted with his drinking. He tries to shift the blame onto me. He starts to bring up an issue he knows will spark an emotional reaction, my failed attempts at applying for positions in my company. He maintains that it is my tarnished past that has kept me from being hired for the positions. For once, I am too tired to fight; I have no emotional reaction. His accusations only add support to my decision to separate.

We pull into the driveway of our rented home and go inside. Joe continues trying to get an emotional reaction from me.

When he doesn't get the reaction he wants he starts toward the door with the car keys in his hand.

I stop him, "Where are you going?"

He tells me he wants to go visit a friend.

"I will drive you there. I don't want you driving the car drunk."

He starts to mock me and call me his mommy for wanting to drive him to his friend's.

I know a fight will develop if I stay, and I am too tired and unsure of my own reaction to stick around for the results. I go into my bedroom, get my purse and head out the door myself. I get into the car, put the keys in the ignition and start it. I look up to see Joe standing in front of the car with a shotgun pointed at me through the windshield. I had been reading books about people who had had guns pointed at them, and I wondered why they just didn't just take off, so that's what I do. I put the car in gear, and pull out of our driveway.

I feel and hear something hit the back of the car. I think Joe has thrown a rock at it. It hurts to think he would throw something at me. Tears start to fill my eyes then run down my face. I head down the road not sure where I am going. The friends we have made during our five years in the small town of Sumas, Washington use alcohol without difficulty. I don't feel they will understand my position. My only other choice is my workplace.

I pull into the lot and find a parking space in front of the office. I get out of the car and walk around to the trunk to see what damage has been caused. I am shocked and hurt to see the shotgun spray on the lower right hand corner of the rear bumper. I go into the office, and when I can't find my supervisor, Bill, I go look for him in the plant.

I find him and the foreman in the plant yard.

"Joe shot the back of the car." I imagine Bill is surprised that I am so calm when I share my news. I'm not sure if I'm in shock or just used to erratic behavior.

Bill tells me I have to call the police.

"No, I can't call the police."

Bill is shocked at my answer and tries to convince me to change my mind by suggesting we ask the police to come to the office first.

Something inside me says that Bill is right, but all I can think about is the cost to me. The money, where will it come from? We are barely scraping by now. How can I take on another financial burden? Calling the authorities will only make things worse, not better. Joe has no way to pay since he has not been working. I will suffer more than he will. However, Bill does have a point. I imagine the authorities coming to the office. I will have the opportunity to tell them about Joe's fragile condition, and maybe things can be handled without too much trouble. I agree to call.

I call the police; the dispatcher keeps me on the phone while she contacts the patrolmen. I can hear the radio in the background and realize things are not going as I had imagined. Rather, the officers are going straight to our house. Joe calls the office on the other line; I put the dispatcher on hold.

"Joe, I called the police."

He is very upset. He can't understand why I did such a thing.

"You shot the back of the car. I had to call the police."

I can tell he is shocked and afraid. He hangs up, and I go back to the dispatcher on the other line.

Shortly after, a neighbor pulls up outside the office with our eight-year-old son. Joe asked the neighbor to bring him to me. I wasn't concerned about his safety because I know Joe wouldn't harm him. I figure Joe must be expecting trouble, or he wouldn't have sent my son to me.

Over the telephone receiver I can hear a person on the radio say that the neighbor has heard several gunshots. I am certain, Joe has committed suicide.

I go into hysterical sobbing as I think about what I am hearing.

I repeat, "What will I do if he has committed suicide? It will be my fault. I don't know if I can take it."

There are several more uncertain minutes before the dispatcher comes back and tells me Joe is in custody.

In Washington, the state brings charges against the suspect in domestic violence cases. I don't know if I could have brought charges against him if it had been up to me.

For the following weeks I let circumstances determine each step I took. Bill told me that I could take some time off. The elementary school was out for spring break, so I decided to take the week off and drive to Utah. When Bill's wife called to offer support, I told her that I wished she could go with me, because I worried about driving the one thousand miles alone with my son, (I tend to get sleepy while driving long distances). She hung up the phone then called right back to tell me that Bill would ride with me rather than fly to the business meeting he was attending in Salt Lake City, Utah. I thankfully accepted the offer, but felt that it was quite a sacrifice. Because Bill was on a business trip, the company paid for the gas. I was able to drive the entire distance without difficulty, but it was reassuring to know I had a backup just in case I became sleepy.

In Salt Lake City I went to my employer's main office. Within the first half-hour, five people approached me and asked if I had applied for the position in graphics. It was starting to look like someone was trying to tell me something. I arranged for an interview. In the interview, the supervisor, Jay offered me the job. I didn't accept. Rather, I told him what had happened. I told him that I had to talk to Joe before I could accept the position. Jay gave me a week to decide. Each day that week brought me closer to making the decision to take the position and return to Utah. My dad offered to loan me the money it would take to move. But I was still not sure until I walked into work the following Monday. Bill told me that he needed to know what my decision was.

"I'm taking the position in Salt Lake."

Jay needed me as soon as possible. I told him I would be there in two weeks. For those next two weeks I felt like a robot. My friend came by to help pack my belongings. I felt so overwhelmed I couldn't do it. The guys from work rallied and pitched in. They each did what they could to help. My brother flew in from Idaho to help drive the moving van as far as Idaho.

Joe volunteered to be admitted to a treatment facility. He was under court order to not contact me.

As soon as I returned from my trip to Utah, I called the treatment facility and asked to talk to Joe. They kept the court order and would not let me talk to him.

"I need to tell him I'm moving back to Salt Lake City in two weeks."

The counselor agreed to give Joe the message.

In the two weeks before our move to Utah, my children and I attended the family treatment program offered at the treatment facility. At the facility, one counselor changed her conviction of not giving recommendations to patients and told me to take my children and run.

I knew the counselor was only trying to help. I did pack up my children and leave, but with the intention of allowing Joe to join us after he served his sentence of three months in treatment and two weeks in jail. I warned him that if he drank or took drugs again our marriage would be over.

# Chapter 2

## I Needed Recovery Too

*Thankfully my Higher Power put me in front of a mirror and told me to take a good look. It was eye opening to realize that I was not in a position to make a judgement.*

I didn't think running from my problems would solve them. The truth was, I needed recovery too. But what were my options? They were:

**1. I could separate from the addict.**

I knew that leaving Joe wasn't the answer for me. I knew that without recovery myself, I would turn around and draw someone just like him. It had been a regular pattern for me all of my life.

**2. I could send the addict to treatment.**

Early in our relationship I called the employee assistance program offered through the company where I worked. The program representative gave me the names of area treatment facilities, for my addict husband. That bit of advice did nothing for me, but offer false hope. The shooting incident did cause Joe to start his successful recovery, but what about my recovery? At the time I didn't know if his recovery would be successful, or how it would affect me.

**3. I could join a support group.**

You might think a support group would offer healing and recovery. Maybe it does for some, but I didn't find recovery or healing at Al-Anon. I did attend several meetings with different groups from Utah to Washington. I enjoyed their support, and I do recommend them for support. But I was confused when they told me to stop my unhealthy behavior. Unfortunately, I didn't understand what I was doing, or why I did it, or I would have stopped years ago. My behavior was all I had known my entire life. I was so deep into the dysfunction that I couldn't see beyond it.

**4. I could read all of the books written on co-dependent behavior.**

I didn't think that I was a co-dependent, since I really didn't know what the term co-dependent meant. Why would I choose to read those books?

None of the four choices listed above were the answer for me. Yet, in my time of need, they seemed to be the only options available. But, none of them offered healing from the inside.

I have found recovery in the nine plus years since the incident and I have experienced tremendous healing. But before I could find health I needed to understand some fundamental truths. As this book proceeds, I will share how I overcame the following ten revelations that have taken years to discover and grasp:

**1. I was contributing to the unhealthy behavior.**

**2. I needed recovery and healing too.**

**3. My own beliefs have prevented me from experiencing joy.**

**4. If I do not feel love for myself, I cannot give love.**

**5. I have the power to change beliefs that no longer work for me.**

**6. My thoughts create my experiences.**

**7. I have total control of my thoughts.**

**8. I have no control over the actions of others.**

**9. Everything works together for a purpose.**

**10. Discomfort does not go away, it becomes an adventure.**

Even though it has been many years since my desperate calls to the company's employee assistance program, I don't think the advice offered has changed. If I called today I would probably get the same advice;

find a way to sober up your addict and your problems will be solved.

When my husband and I look back at the incident, we realize that the painful events were necessary to bring us to the subsequent nine years of clean and sober life. I still feel sorrow every time I think of my husband pointing a gun at me. My husband is horrified to think that during a drunken blackout he came that close to harming the most important person in his life. But without the experience, I would not have found the recovery and healing I needed.

My recovery began when I started to accept responsibility. Once I accepted responsibility, an overall plan became apparent, and once I understood the concept of an overall plan, the blame disappeared. These realizations lead me to start seeing my experiences as opportunities to learn and grow.

I just didn't automatically start accepting responsibility. I had to make a change inside of me. I had to change my perception. This change in perception was my first clue that lasting peace, joy and happiness were dependent on internal change, rather than the external change I had been praying for. I wasn't alone in the belief that peace, joy and happiness can be found through external pleasures. It is promoted by our culture. Advertisements have shown us that if we are unhappy we can turn to an outside substance to make us feel better. Some of us might choose to eat a piece of chocolate to improve our disposition. Others look to a drug or an alcoholic beverage to find their happiness. We can watch television to see how these various external substances affect others. The people in the commercials are beautiful, and they always look happy.

With internal change in perception, I found that the external is not eternal, and the happiness we find is short lived. If we fill our lives with external pleasures, two things can happen: 1) we can neglect our internal needs by substituting them with external pleasures, 2) we can start to believe we are in control, as we manipulate the external inanimate objects.

I'm not suggesting that we stop enjoying external pleasures. When we pamper ourselves we are showing ourselves love. It's just that external pleasures cannot offer lasting inner peace, joy and happiness.

With awareness, we have control over our internal wellbeing or dysfunction. Our internal condition will cause us to draw like-kind external circumstances. Our external circumstances become a mirror of our internal condition. If we are experiencing internal wellbeing, we will draw similar external wellbeing circumstances. In the same way, internal dysfunction will draw similar external dysfunctional circumstances. This concept is explained in John and Linda Friel's book, *Adult Children, The Secrets of Dysfunctional Families.* The Friels believe that two healthy people will draw to one another, and in the same way two unhealthy people will draw to one another.

We draw to us what is familiar (internal condition draws external replication). We look for what we know and what feels comfortable to us. Two mountain climbers might meet, get married and live happily ever after climbing mountains together. And in the same way two unhealthy people might meet one another and live together unhealthily. As with Joe and me, we grew up with similar types of signals: "Don't talk, don't feel and don't trust." Therefore, we drew to one another (I'll share more about the similarities in Chapter 3). If all we know is unhappiness, we will draw someone who will give us that familiar experience.

There is a reason why we draw external replication. It is to help us learn and grow. Our spiritual self will bring a reflection of our internal beliefs by way of external experiences. Those external likes and dislikes are there to help us identify our internal likes and dislikes. Reflections are a great tool. When we identify how we feel about ourselves, we can change the beliefs that don't work to our benefit. Don't forget that reflections are not there for judgement or blame. They are our teachers to aid in our growth, development and recovery.

I didn't understand the true value of reflection as a tool. For the nine plus years prior to my husband's sobriety, I had been under the impression that I could discover peace by changing my external circumstances (I was going about it backwards). It took my addict finding sobriety before I realized my error. With his sobriety, my external circumstances had changed. When inner peace didn't automatically follow, I had to look further to find it. I could no longer blame him. I had to accept responsibility for my part in the dysfunction. With acceptance of responsibility, I discovered four powerful truths. 1. I experienced tremendous release (the opposite of what I had imagined). 2. I could move past the belief that my external experiences were responsible for my peace, joy and happiness. 3. By examining my reflections, I could see what internal changes I needed to make. 4. I alone held the key to my happiness.

With my new understanding of reflections, I could see how important it would be for me to discover self-love. According to what I had learned, if I loved myself, I would draw love into my life. Loving me had not been a part of my life for many years. I discovered that with a few internal thought process changes, I could rediscover self-love.

Self-love hadn't been a part of my life because over the years I had established some disabling beliefs about myself. I could pinpoint some of those beliefs. I believed that I was unworthy. According to my religious teachings, I had sinned. I believed I was unlovable. I don't remember the first time I heard the words "I love you," but it was late into my twenties. I believed I was not deserving. Sinners do not deserve happiness. By nurturing these beliefs about myself, I was drawing the external circumstances in my life that proved me right. In addition, I was denying myself the abundant gifts offered by a gracious Universe.

In order to find self-love, I had to change the known beliefs mentioned above and uncover and change any others that were hidden. If I did not have love for myself, I could not give true love to others.

It took my addict getting sober, for my journey toward self-love to begin. My external circumstances had to change before I could experience the difference between external satisfaction and the fullness of internal peace.

Finding inner peace is not subject to an external change. Others may not need an external change as I did to realize the importance of self-love. After we find inner peace our reflections will change. We will draw to ourselves like-kind external circumstances, as explained earlier in this chapter.

I know it all sounds simple, because it is simple. We can change our life by learning how to nurture ourselves inside. Our life will not be free of discomfort after we find self-love. We might think we want a comfortable life. But if we had a comfortable life, we would stop learning and growing. It is the discomfort that teaches all of us our grandest lessons. Once we start to see the value of discomfort, we can embrace it as an adventure and see it as a new opportunity for growth.

For many years I didn't see my discomfort as an adventure. I was in denial. I wanted my external circumstances to change. My addict was the problem. Consequently, I didn't want to change anything that I was doing. But once I found that I could gain peace, joy and happiness through taking responsibility, I wanted further healing and recovery. To gain further healing and recovery, I needed to understand more about the disease and how it affected my family and me.

# Chapter 3

## Families and Substance Abuse

*The Recovery Center realized that without the help and support of the friends and family members, the chance for long-term recovery was lessened. They also recognized that the family members were or had become, as toxic as the substance-addict was.*

I learned about the "don't talk, don't feel, don't trust" behaviors mentioned in Chapter 2, at the treatment facility my husband checked in to, two separate times. The first time in 1988, I convinced Joe to check himself into The Recovery Center at St. Joseph

Hospital in Bellingham Washington, for the treatment of his alcoholism and drug addiction. As a part of the treatment, the family members were encouraged, even bribed, to attend the family program at The Recovery Center facility. If the friends and family members came to treatment on Thursday, Friday and Saturday, they could join their substance-addict for dinner at the center on Sunday.

The Recovery Center realized that without the help and support of the friends and family members, the chance for long-term recovery was lessened. They also recognized that the family members were or had become, as toxic as the substance-addict was.

The Recovery Center compared the substance-addict and the relationship with his/her family, to a mobile. If one item on the mobile moves, the other items move to counter balance the motion. In the same respect, in the family of the substance-addict, the substance-addict acts out, and the family members react.

Many times, specific roles are created in the family of the substance-addict to survive the inconsistent and many times chaotic behavior. The role-players have two sets of feelings: those they experience inside and a second set they present to the outside.

**The Drug Addict or Alcoholic** is the chemically dependent family member.

Inner feelings: guilt, shame and self-hate

Outward feelings: anger, accusing and righteousness

**The Chief Enabler** is the person in charge, the one the substance-addict is most dependent upon. As the substance-addict loses control, the chief enabler takes over his or her responsibilities.

Inner feelings: anger, fear and guilt

Outward feelings: self-pity, super responsibility and manipulation

**The Family Hero** is the individual who provides the family's self-worth.

Inner feelings: loneliness, hurt and inadequacy

Outward feelings: success and approval seeking

**The Scapegoat** is the one distracting the focus of the family's attention, usually in destructive ways. This family member has learned that it's not who you are, but what you do which matters.

Inner feelings: loneliness, rejection and anger

Outward feelings: defiance and acting out, this individual may start to use addictive behaviors, drugs or alcohol.

**The Invisible Child** offers relief, by being good.

Inner feelings: pain, loneliness and anger

Outward feelings: quietness, independence

**The Clown's** contribution is with fun and humor.

Inner feelings: confusion and insecurity

Outward feelings: making light of matters

As I write, my family is in its tenth year of recovery. The health that has accompanied those recovery years is remarkable and very noticeable after living with toxicity for over nine years. Before recovery, my attachment to my husband meant that I lived in fear that he would make a decision that would cause me to suffer consequences. With that attachment, I had given up control over my own life. I was so immersed in my husband's addiction, that I had no time to nurture myself. I spent much of my time pointing my finger in judgement and blame rather that going within to find the healing I required. Now that alcohol and drugs are no longer an all-consuming part of our lives, we have the time and energy to go within to find inner healing.

(Many families outside of drug addiction and alcoholism may practice the roles mentioned earlier. But without the disease, they are not pronounced and therefore not as noticeable.)

We learned in the treatment program that the substance-addicts and their families need to recognize situations that can trigger the need to find comfort in a substance. One effective acronym is the word HALT, if we are "H" hungry, "A" angry, "L" lonely or "T" tired, we need to take immediate action to satisfy one or all of these needs.

The Recovery Center recognized the need to support and encourage the friends and family members. In some treatment facilities, the friends and family members are not included in the treatment program. The absence of family education could be attributed to the misunderstanding of the disease in our culture. Many still believe that the problem of substance abuse is a matter of willpower. If willpower were the answer, this country would not have 11 million plus individuals struggling in the disease. Lack of funding could also be the reason why facilities don't include family members in the treatment. Therapy is costly. But if we can prevent further dysfunction, the future costs to society could be greatly reduced. If we don't believe that substance abuse is a social problem, we only need to watch the television program *Cops*. I don't remember ever seeing a person being arrested on the show that was not under the influence of a substance. Experts in the field of substance abuse are still working on how to best treat the disease of substance abuse.

The Recovery Center focused the time set aside for friends and family members to inform through education. As I mentioned earlier, the family members were encouraged to come to family treatment therapy every Thursday, Friday, Saturday and Sunday during the twenty-one-day program. Our treatment consisted of group discussions where we could talk about how we felt. Counselors facilitated these sessions and were available to help if the friends and family members needed further understanding. Joint classes were offered where my family and my husband learned more about the disease of substance-addiction. On Sundays special guests were invited to share how substance-addiction had affected their lives. Through all of these sessions we learned that substance-addiction is a family disease. On average the substance-addict affects the lives of <u>four</u> other people. I have learned this to be true in my family's experience with our substance-addict.

In addition to gaining help through treatment centers, my children and I were introduced to various support groups. The twelve-step program for me is Al-Anon. My children can attend COA, children of alcoholics. Al-Anon and COA are groups where friends and family members can find support from others with similar experiences.

No wimps allowed! I found with the Al-Anon groups that I attended. The other participants would not allow members to continue to play the victim. Seasoned Al-Anon veterans told me to discontinue my unhealthy behavior. Unfortunately, I was so deep in the dysfunction that I didn't know what was unhealthy behavior. I needed more than being told to simply stop. This behavior was my life; it was all I knew how to do. The truth was, I needed a recovery program that would help me to understand my behavior.

With understanding we can go inside to find our own truths, learn who we are, and accept with confidence that we are exactly what we need to be, and that our experiences are what made us the unique wonderful individual we are today. With this new confidence we will discover that our decisions come from our heart, and are not disputed by those around us. And, we will draw people to us whose wellbeing is equal to ours. No victims please, heal and move on.

# Chapter 4

## The Disease

*"An alcoholic looks good on the outside, yet is a total wreck on the inside."*

*Joe Ehrler*

I have often said it wasn't the actual drinking that bothered me about my husband, it was his behavior. Joe hated himself so much that he subconsciously and consciously tried to project some of that self-hate, guilt and shame onto those who were closest to him.

I use the term addict in this book, because to me the term fits Joe's condition. He was powerless over alcohol and drugs. Many experts no longer use the term addict. Substance abuser or dependent, are terms that more clearly define a disease that is diverse in its effect on its victims. An individual can abuse a substance and not be addicted. An individual dependent on a substance will experience withdrawal or craving because he/she is physiologically or psychologically dependent on the substance. Many individuals drink socially. When an individual continues to use a substance despite negative legal or social consequences, most experts in the field of alcohol and drug treatment would agree that they are abusing that substance.

Another misunderstood term in the field of substance abuse is blackout. Many confuse it with the term passed-out. When in fact, during a substance-induced blackout, the individual is functioning with all his or her faculties (in an intoxicated state). But the individual has no memory of their actions or the events that took place during the blackout.

In *The Addictive Personality*, Craig Nakken writes that addicts use objects in an effort to change the natural ups and downs of life. The addict starts to rely on outside objects to experience a change in his/her mood. Addiction is a progressive disease. In the case of alcohol or drug addiction, the addict establishes an emotional attachment to the substance, using it to delay uncomfortable issues. The substance starts to replace the need for human interaction. The substance becomes the first choice, leaving human interaction as a second choice. The relationship of the addict to the object is destructive and unnatural. Natural relationships include friends and family, spiritual Higher Power, self and community. The relationship to the substance is predictable in the beginning, where relationships with others are not predictable.

John and Linda Friel suggest in their book, *Adult Children, The Secrets of Dysfunctional Families*, that there are social/emotional factors that are common to addictive agents. In the case of the alcohol or drug addict the addictive agent is the substance. The social/emotional factors are:

1. *Temporary anxiety reduction.*
2. *Temporary stress reduction.*
3. *Temporary feelings of power and wellbeing.*
4. *Avoidance of true feelings.*
5. *Avoidance of crucial problems and developmental tasks.*
6. *Avoidance of intimacy.*

While in treatment at the Recovery Center, we were told that an alcoholic suppresses a year of emotional growth each year that he/she drinks. Emotional issues are drowned in an alcohol-induced or drug-enhanced stupor, rather than dealt with as they arise. Joe is still making up time after twenty-seven years of drinking. As they say in AA, alcoholism is a cunning, powerful and baffling disease. I do believe addiction is a disease. I watched Joe absorbed in regret and self-hate, making promises to never touch another drop, only to be caught in the grip of dependence hours later.

Both Joe and I thought that he would have to die before he could quit drinking. I figured that I would have to be the one to watch him do so. I'm thankful that both of us started to realize that we needed help.

We've come to realize that the addict in our lives is living under a different set of rules. As Craig Nakken writes about the addictive cycle:

> *Any addiction relationship begins when a person repeatedly seeks the illusion of relief to avoid unpleasant feelings or situations. This is nurturing through avoidance—an unnatural way of taking care of one's emotional needs. At this point, addicts start to give up natural relationships and the relief they offer.*

And again Nakken writes about the addictive personality:

> *This personality does not exist prior to the illness of addiction, nor does it represent a predisposition to addiction; rather it emerges from the addictive process....The addict side of the personality is very important for the recovering addicts to understand because it will stay with them for life.*

Based on Nakken's findings, even after treatment, our addict will still be living with an altered personality. Through understanding, we can make the healthy decision to accept and detach from our addict. We probably do not like that our practicing alcoholic is in self-destruction mode, but we can do nothing to change that fact. Only the alcoholic can choose recovery. Physiology may impact the ability of the addict to make that decision.

Many experts believe the disease is inherited. My father-in-law was an alcoholic. I didn't know him because he died on Christmas day in 1979. His death was caused from the injuries he sustained after falling down a flight of stairs a few days earlier. He was drunk at the time. According to my husband, his grandfather was also an alcoholic. A publication of the National Clearinghouse for Alcohol and Drug Information reported there was an estimated 28.6 million children of alcoholics in the United States in 1991. These high numbers might sound frightening to the loved ones of the substance-addicted. But the good news is that more is being learned about genetics and the disease of alcoholism. It is in this area where prevention education can substantially effect outcome.

I do not believe that everyone who drinks has a drinking problem. Individuals in recovery refer to social drinkers as 'normies'. Even though I can be classified as a 'normie', I rarely drink, and when I do it is in small amounts. In my family, drinking was a problem that has caused much pain. I have no desire to recreate the unhappiness.

It took me many years to learn that I could not force my addict to choose recovery. In the process, I also learned that there are no defined "do's and don'ts" on how to interact with the addict in our lives. In the following paragraphs I will explain: that we can have non-judgement; we can understand that the beliefs of others can effect whether our addict chooses recovery; we can learn to accept the lessons: ours and theirs; and we can give our support. I know practicing non-judgement sounds like something we are doing for our addict, but in truth, judgement is devastating to our internal wellbeing. When we have judgement of others, we usually have judgement of ourselves. Acceptance of self is a major goal as we seek inner recovery and healing.

In addition, if we judge our addict's behavior, we will not change our addict; we will only bring feelings of guilt, regret and shame. In the same respect, we should not judge ourselves for our failure to be conscious of our unhealthy behavior.

There is a commonly held belief that an addict is someone out of control, living on the streets, panhandling, walking around with a bottle in a brown paper bag and sleeping it off on a park bench. This belief can alienate the addict who appears to have it all together, yet may need help.

Since the addict's primary relationship is with an object, the friends and family members of the addict are left trying to understand someone who has placed the nurturing of people second to their substance.

We can't take the life lessons away from our loved ones, no matter how much we would like to do so. If we do step in and rescue them, they will have to make up that essential lesson in one way or another, and the lesson might be harder the next time. We believe and trust in our own Higher Power as knowing what is best for us. In the same way, we can trust that the Higher

Power of our loved one is helping them through the life they need to live, even if it isn't according to our idea of what should be.

Our lessons can be difficult. If we find ourselves in a situation that feels too burdensome for us to handle, we can get quiet and ask our Higher Power what lesson we need to learn. We can open our heart and hear the answer, ask for strength and trust that we are supported. There is always professional help if we feel we need it.

What can we do to help those around us if we can't control them? We can give them our support.

I attended a seminar sponsored by the company I worked for. It was a ropes-course, a term used to describe the physical activity such as climbing poles and balancing on tightropes. For the course we split into several groups. Each group worked together as a team. When one member of the team was performing a ropes-course activity, it was the job of the others in the team to support their team member. In essence, a cheerleading squad supported every member. I was a better cheerleader than pole climber.

The first day was spent performing physical activities. The tone was so casual, and the support so rampant that my teammate congratulated the Human Resource manager with a slap to the backside. The tone was non-judgement, anything goes, and we are all in this together.

The next day was spent in the classroom, dancing, hugging and supporting one another. An hour was set aside for individual reflection about our future desires.

We were set loose amongst the stillness and beauty of nature, and encouraged to avoid contact with other humans while we reflected. After the hour was up, I realized that if I had the support and encouragement I had experienced while at the seminar, I would want to stay with the organization offering that type of support.

When I shared my discovery in front of my fellow course-mates uncontrollable audible sobs poured from me. The support continued when the entire first row of seated individuals jumped up to offer support to my emotional announcement. My heart swells just thinking about it.

We went back to the office, and everything went back to the way it had been before we went to the seminar.

Why did everyone climb back into the same box they were encouraged to climb out of at the seminar? The organizational structure of the company had not changed. It was still organized in the pyramid organizational structure. Something at the core needed to change; the pyramid structure is simply not conducive to the teamwork philosophy.

In the same respect, to establish our role of support, each of us might have to change the structure we have established at our core. We can do this by being open to new thought processes, ones that are outside our familiar "box." We might find our structure is not conducive to the support and acceptance needed. But change is necessary if we haven't found the peace that <u>is</u> available to each one of us.

Understanding our behavior and the behavior of those around us can help us to find recovery and healing. I credit my Higher Power for my understanding, healing and recovery. This book and everything in your life comes to you exactly when you need it, brought to you by your Higher Power. And, I have asked my Higher Power to help this book find you. You too can ask and receive. Let's move on to positive and possible life changing truths.

# Chapter 5

## Unlimited, Loving and Gracious Spirit

*The spiritual aspects needed for recovery and healing were always available to my husband and me. But it took us many years before we realized the full spiritual potential available.*

Whenever we are experiencing discomfort, our Higher Power is available to comfort us. Our Higher Power is there to accompany us on our journey toward inner healing. In the Alcoholics Anonymous twelve-step program, the third step is one of the most powerful of the twelve steps. With this step, the participant is encouraged to define their Higher Power in whatever terms they choose, whether it be God, The Universe, The All That Is, the Everywhere Spirit or none of the above.

The recovering substance-addict has learned that identifying with a Higher Power is an effective step toward in his/her successful recovery. Usually by the time the substance-addict finds AA, he/she has tried to stop drinking using his/her will, and he/she has failed many times. The first step of the AA twelve steps encourages the alcoholic to admit he/she is powerless over alcohol. At this point, the alcoholic can choose to find and trust a Higher Power or go back to the uncontrollable life they were living. For the alcoholic or drug addict who desires recovery, the choice becomes an easy one.

My husband, Joe realized the availability of his Higher Power when he asked for help with his substance-addiction. He gives the credit to his Higher Power, for his recovery from the disease of alcoholism and drug addiction. When nothing else worked, he surrendered to his Higher Power. He knows now that everyday he has the support and understanding of his Higher Power. He believes that together they can make it through each day, one day at a time.

In the same way the alcoholic seeks support through their definition of a Higher Power, we can seek the same support using our own definition of our Higher Power. When all of our attempts to find peace have failed, we have one more option. That option is to turn to our Higher Power, which can be defined in the simplest of terms. Some of us might have an unfavorable perception based on some of the terms used to define Higher Power. This was the case with me, the term God brought images of a judgmental Creator anxious to punish sinners. Because this mental picture was no longer my truth, I needed to find a term that brought up images of love and compassion, because those are the characteristics I found my Creator to possess. Sometimes the definition of a term was one we've grown up believing to be true, when in fact the term was not based on our own understanding, but rather on the understanding of others.

Our spiritual experience is between our Higher Power and us. Once we understand this relationship and know we are very capable of having a close relationship with our Higher Power, we will find we have much more available to us than we could have imagined in our wildest dreams.

We can have this relationship with our Higher Power in the privacy of our own home, in our car and even at work. We don't have to do anything, but believe to obtain it, and the love that comes is many times greater than the effort required.

Once I started to rely on my Higher Power, I realized there was much more to it than I could have ever imagined. I found that my Higher Power was not only available to help me find recovery and healing, but that it was an unlimited, loving and gracious resource. With this discovery, I also realized my Higher Power had always been available to me, but that I was the one keeping that resource from me. It was my Higher Power who taught me that judgement was nonexistent. If we as humans can love our children unconditionally, then we must know our Creator has at least that capacity for love and much more. As you can imagine, I wanted to share what I had learned about my Higher Power and spiritual aspects with everyone. In this chapter and for the rest of the book, I am going to do just that.

When I refer to the spiritual, I am not talking about religion, although many people regard the two as the same. Religion is an organized belief of a group of individuals, while spiritual is an individual experience with our Higher Power.

A scientist might disagree with me when I say, there are many truths in this world based on spiritual experiences. Science measures results based on what we smell, touch, hear, taste or see. We have all had experiences outside our five senses that are unexplained scientifically, yet we know in our heart, they are true. If we base everything we know on our five senses then we would have to say the earth is flat and standing still, and the sun is revolving around the earth because that's how it <u>feels</u> and <u>looks</u> to us.

The belief of life after death has not been measured or proven scientifically, yet many of us have embraced it. If we can believe in life after death and a Higher Power, we can go a step further to find the peace, joy and happiness, which is not based on external stimulus, but on inner knowing.

Since the spiritual can't be measured, I have had to trust my inner knowing together with prompting from my Higher Power. This book is written from the heart and based on that trust. My Higher Power always leads me to find my personal highest good, as does yours. For many years I didn't trust and accept the loving support offered by my Higher Power. I mistakenly thought my Higher Power was only available through religion. Even so, contact with my Higher Power wasn't at the personal level. I believed I could talk to my Higher Power through prayer, but the prayers I learned were rehearsed and generic. I did not believe my Higher Power was available on a personal level. In fact, I believed that only powerful church officials could get the Higher Power to answer prayers. The Higher Power I grew up with was judgmental—-sinners were punished.

The Higher Power I knew growing up was too important for the average individual and definitely unavailable to sinners, of which I was one. These beliefs were imprinted. For many years my own beliefs prevented me from experiencing the loving support of my Higher Power, available to all of us. My beliefs were so buried that it has taken several years to locate and change them to beliefs closer to my truth. My new beliefs include an all-powerful, all-knowing Higher Power who is small enough to care for, guide and love each of us individually. My Higher Power now has the ability to comfort me at any moment with unlimited love and caring. I can imagine myself enveloped within the loving energy of my Higher Power. I can feel my Higher Power's love and acceptance of me.

You can see how my beliefs put self-imposed limitations on the availability of my Higher Power. I didn't learn until later in life that my Higher Power is totally supportive of my needs and desires and is anxious to help me find inner peace. To experience this loving support system at anytime and any place, I needed to reexamine the beliefs that were hindering the millions of possibilities and probabilities available through my Higher Power. I needed to replace those disabling beliefs with the truth that I am not alone and never have been.

For many years I believed that I was unworthy, unlovable and not deserving. I was certain that I was a sinner. Who wants to acknowledge a sinner? Especially not my Higher Power. In fact, I believed that I really should have been hiding from my Higher Power. I could have been struck down at any moment! I knew my Higher Power was displeased because my prayers were never answered.

Sound familiar? Many of us might remember a time when we prayed for something and did not get what we wanted. We could be asking for the wrong thing, as I did by asking my Higher Power to change my external circumstances. Not only did I ask for my answer in the wrong way, I prevented my Creator from answering any of my prayers, because I had some powerful disabling beliefs (that I was unlovable, unworthy and not deserving). When we can start to:

1. **Transmute disabling beliefs.**
2. **Understand and believe that we each have unlimited access to a giving Universe.**
3. **Realize that we learn by living through uncomfortable experiences.**

Our pathway to know our Higher Power becomes paved and open to traffic. I learned that our Higher Power is available and anxious to answer our prayers.

After hearing my spiel on thinking positively and receiving answers to prayers, a friend reminded me that our physical bodies have limitations. He gave the example that as a child he wanted to fly. He said he truly believed he could fly, and he prayed to be able to do so. But no matter how hard he flapped his arms, he could not lift off of the ground. I had just read all three books by Robert Monroe on OBE (out of the body experiences). According to Monroe, one can fly, but when using OBE, they have to leave their body behind. In addition, many of us have flown in our dreams (another form of OBE), and let's not forget airplanes.

When I shared the OBE possibility with my friend, he wasn't very receptive to the idea. It's possible that I planted a seed that will help him to accept the out of the body flying when his prayers are answered, and he finds himself on the ceiling looking down at his body. OBE is a difficult concept to accept and whether we choose to believe in it or not is irrelevant. I think my friend has received an answer to prayer if he has flown in an airplane. It's just that his answer didn't come in the way or the time frame he expected.

(There are many stories about saints and spiritual masters being able to levitate and even fly physically. I believe we are truly without limits, but the answer is within, not outside us.)

I had another friend who shared a painful childhood experience regarding sexual abuse; she learned to let her mind wander into space during the assault. Belief in God is not a part of her life because she believed her prayers were requested, but not answered. I told her that her prayer was answered. She was given the ability to mentally leave her body during the unpleasant experience. And, the abuse did stop, once she grew up. I'm certainly not condoning the behavior, but we cannot change our past experiences. I recommend professional therapy for anyone who has experienced this type of abuse. In addition to therapy, we can decide to change the way we view our experiences. We can choose to be traumatized and forsake God, or we can look for the growth experience and know that there is a master plan. With professional help and changed perception we can go on to offer support to others because we experienced how it feels.

Our High Power will help us to make the permanent changes that must come from the inside. Internal health can be discovered when we:

**1. Become aware of our internal wellbeing or dysfunction.**

- **Take Responsibility.**
- **Without blame and judgement**

**2. Change our perception.**

- **Understand the universal plan.**
- **Accept and celebrate life experiences.**
- **Thank Higher Power for its gracious gift of life.**

**3. Discover self-love.**

- **Recite affirmations.**

- **Discover disabling beliefs.**
- **Change beliefs that no longer are of value.**

In the chart following this page and through the next three chapters, I will share with you the process I discovered that led me to the peace, joy and happiness I experience today.

## Recovery and Healing; It's an Inside Job

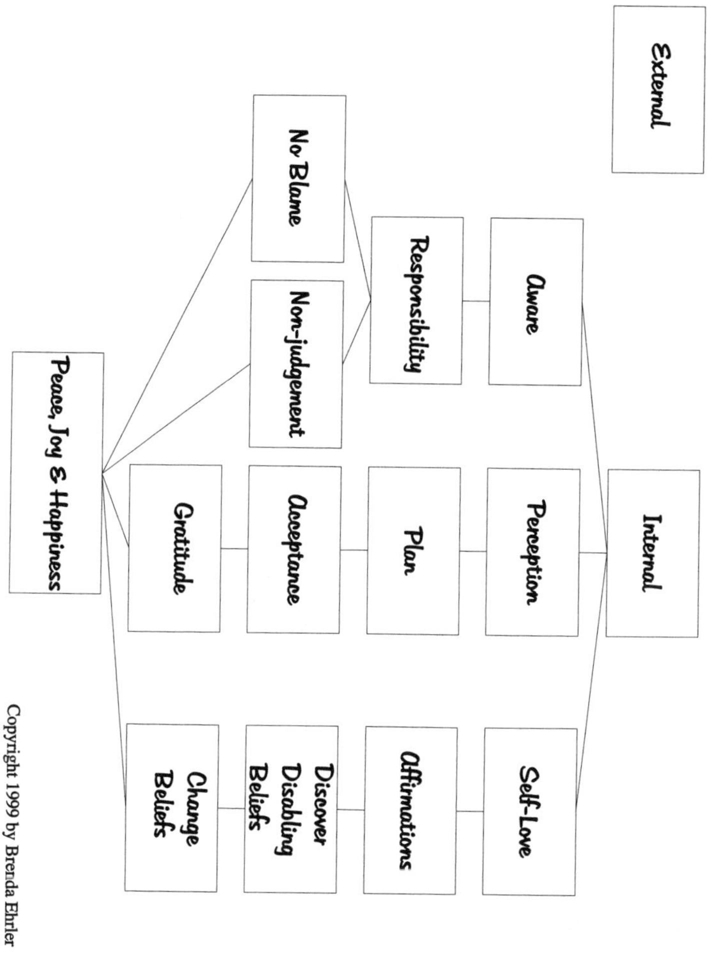

# Chapter 6

## Becoming Aware and Taking Responsibility

*Webster's New World dictionary defines dysfunction as: Abnormal, impaired, or incomplete functioning, as of a body organ or part.*

I struggled with the term dysfunctional because when I heard the word I pictured blame, judgement and comparison of one human to another. You'll notice as you read this book that I'm opposed to blame, judgement and comparison. I felt as though I needed to use the word dysfunction, but there seemed to be a contradiction. In the following paragraphs I am going to attempt to justify the use of the word in this book and change our perception of the word dysfunction.

Let's look at the word not as a comparison of one person's behavior to that of another, but to evaluate how the behavior of a part affects that of the whole. Stay with me and consider the following points:

**The dysfunctional part of the body**. If our liver were not functioning, the health of our body would be affected. We could die. We do not blame, judge or compare the liver. We just want to find a way to bring it back to health.

**The dysfunctional part in relationship to our family as a whole**. The emotional health and wellbeing of our immediate family is important. We need the stability and support at the family level, for each family member to take confidence and security out into the world of work, play and school. If one family member is functioning in a way that is detrimental to the health of our family unit, we want to find a way to bring the family unit back to health. We would not use blame, judgement or comparison to repair the family unit. Those tactics would only further the dysfunction through alienation and separation. Rather, we would choose support and understanding.

I use the term dysfunctional in an effort to bring light and understanding to something that needs attention without using blame, judgement or comparison. According to John Friel and Linda Friel in their book, *Adult Children, The Secrets of Dysfunctional Families*, 90 to 95 percent of the population are practicing some form of dysfunction.

That's a lot of dysfunction. If we were to continue to deal with dysfunction by using blame, judgement and comparison, we could live for many years missing the point. An example would be me blaming my husband and holding him responsible for my joy for nine years. I asked God more than once to help my husband find sobriety so that I could be happy. I judged him as guilty for bringing unhappiness into my life. Thankfully my Higher Power put me in front of a mirror, and told me to take a good look. It was eye opening to realize that I was not in a position to make a judgement. This was my first step in realizing that I needed to focus on bringing light to my dysfunction (without blame, judgement or comparison) before I could begin to find joy in my life.

As we bring our dysfunction to light, we must remember there should be no judgement, for judgement will not lead to healing. To the contrary, when we make a judgement blaming ourselves, our parents, our siblings or even the bully from our grade school, we are so busy pointing our finger that we quit working on our own internal recovery and healing.

If we were to try to find blame for dysfunction, we would have to go back to the beginning of time. We act because of our experiences, and our beliefs, as did our parents and their parents before them, and their parents before them, and so on and so on. It is the accumulation of all of our actions that make us who we are today. If we are not happy with ourselves, blame and judgement of our past will only add to our displeasure. Understanding more about my dysfunction helped me in my healing process.

The Friels helped to define what may have caused some of my dysfunction in their book, *Adult Children, The Secrets of Dysfunctional Families*. They write.

> *The family has several functions that it serves, just as any other system has functions. Many of these functions meet family members' needs. For example, there are maintenance functions, in which basic needs such as food, clothing and shelter are met. When the furnace breaks down someone fixes it. When we outgrow our clothes, someone provides new ones. When we are hungry, someone feeds us.*

According to the Friel's definition of basic needs I received food, clothing, shelter, safety and warmth. I received the basic needs from my family, but the nurturing was missing. My mother was 39 years old when I was born. From what I remember, she suffered from depression for much of her adult life. She didn't have enough energy to give nurturance to herself, let alone to a family that included a newborn.

In our family, it was regular behavior not to show affection to one another. The Friel's would consider this type of behavior, dysfunctional. As a youngster, I remember watching with curiosity, my best friend and her dad. They always kissed hello and goodbye. My friend could easily show affection. She was able to do so with my dad. She seemed to bring out the best in him. Whenever my dad saw her, he smiled and accepted her affection. He would call out his pet name for her, open his arms up and hug her thin body close to his. After witnessing all of this affection, I surprised my dad with a kiss, but I didn't like the feeling. The kiss felt cold and hard (like a stone wall). I understand now that this lack of affection did not mean that we didn't love one another. Neither one of us knew how to comfortably show physical affection to family members.

At that young age, I was not upset that my friend got the hugs rather than me. I was glad my dad showed her the extra affection. Being raised with none, I figured he did it because he loved her as much as I did. It wasn't until later in life that I felt a bit envious of my friend for being bold enough to give and take affection. My friend wasn't the only outsider my dad was able to open up to. Outside our home he was a very gregarious man. It was easy for him to show genuine affection to the people he knew, but not to his own family.

When he passed away, my brother and I were standing by his casket at the viewing, greeting his friends and family members. A distant relative of ours looked at dad's body and shared that he looked good, but his familiar smile was missing. My brother and I looked at one another. I was the first to ask, "What smile?" I don't blame dad. He was only doing what he had learned from his parents. The story helps me to understand why I drew an alcoholic into my life. An alcoholic would offer the solitude that I grew up with. These experiences had become comfortable to me. My dad's sister shared that they were taught to not build up their children for fear that they might become over-confident. I guess humble rather than confident children were the fashion when they were growing up in the early 1900's.

Many of us come from families that are unable to show love and this may be one reason dysfunctional behavior continues. I did not delve into my past, so that I could place blame onto others. I did so to help further understanding. With awareness we can stop the dysfunctional behavior we are practicing. As I mentioned earlier, my dysfunction drew me to an alcoholic/drug addict. This action led us to a substance abuse treatment center. At the treatment center we learned about behaviors and roles identified in the family members of the substance-addict.

Becoming aware can help us as we discover what we need for recovery. We can further enhance our journey with a support group. If one group doesn't feel right, try another. At Al-Anon, you will have someone with similar experiences to share your feelings with. Be aware that looking in the mirror can be painful.

My ongoing recovery was dependent on becoming aware of my behavior. Through awareness, I started to realize that my actions were just reactions to those around me, I didn't know who I was! As you read earlier, I believed that if I could change the lives of those around me, I could find happiness. Before I could stop acting out in dysfunctional ways, I needed to learn more about me, not the reacting person that I had become. I feared looking at the person I had become. I have had to dig deep to discover feelings. I'm continually realizing just how little I know about me. There are many others like me, individuals who don't understand what makes their actions so dysfunctional.

Awareness will help us on our journey to find inner self-love. With inner self-love our reactions will change and will be based on confidence and truth rather than emotion and fear. With awareness, we can uncover some of our disabling beliefs, examine and change them into positive beliefs (we will discuss more about self-love and beliefs in Chapter 8). When we change ourselves inside, our new attitude and the resulting shift in behaviors bring change in the people around us. In some cases, the people in our lives go away, and in some cases their behavior changes. Through changing our hearts, we can change our situations no matter what they are.

In the following paragraphs I will share my understanding of some of the identified dysfunctional behaviors of the friends and family members of the substance-addicted.

I broke the term co-dependent down to further understand the possible meaning. The prefix "co" means joint. Webster defines dependent as, "influenced, controlled or determined by something else; contingent." If we take the definition literally co-dependent could mean that the substance jointly controls us along with our substance-addict. Or we could be jointly dependent on the effects of the substance, perhaps in the same way that our substance-addict turns to drugs or alcohol to control the natural ups and downs of life. The friends and family members use the substance abuse of the addict to try to control the natural ups and downs in their lives. The substance-addict has control over the substance for a time, but then it takes control of him/her. The friend and family member feels as though they are in control, but never have control over the substance-addict's behavior.

(I prefer the terms "friends and family members" or "loved ones" rather than co-dependent. But there are places in this book where I use co-dependent, for lack of a better term.)

When the definitions are unclear for the terms "co-dependent" and "too much", they can be used by others and by us to make judgements of our behaviors. With judgement comes guilt, shame and regret. And, with guilt, shame and regret the dysfunctional cycle starts all over again.

Even with unclear definition, there are behaviors I think most of us would recognize as co-dependent behavior: 1) taking on the responsibility of others, 2) using manipulation to reach a desired end, 3) attempting to control the external events in our life to reach internal peace, 4) attaching financially and emotionally to another individual, 5) enabling an individual to continue unhealthy behavior without recrimination. All of these behaviors are performed with the best of intentions. And many times we practice them simply because it is all we know to do. I needed to become aware and take responsibility for my unhealthy behaviors before I could continue on my path to inner healing and recovery.

**1. Taking on the responsibility of others**

If we are in the role of caregiver, we can feel justified about taking on the responsibility of others. Many times the mothers in our culture tend to give of themselves until their own resources are depleted. The dependent family members become used to the mother who gives and expects nothing in return. This mother/family relationship is accepted, and many times expected in our culture. A mother might measure her worth by the accomplishments of her family.

The message I got when I was growing up was that women were supposed to care for others. I don't remember any training on caring for myself. I guess I would be reaping a benefit by default when I ate the nutritious meal I was learning to prepare for my family in my high school home economics course.

In some cultures women still give of themselves selflessly. Being a selfless mother appears to be the right thing to do on the outside. But these mothers are practicing a disservice to their family. They send a powerful signal to the family members that self is unimportant. Thus, selfless mothers continue the cycle of low self-worth. By example they teach their family that one does not need to care for oneself, but rather that it is their duty to care only for others. A true gift of love must be felt from within first. I was following this practice and taking my son's responsibility in the following example.

At a recent parent-teacher conference, I was at a loss. My 17-year-old was not attending his classes, and when he was there, he was only there physically. While I talked to his first two teachers, my mind was busy trying to figure out how I was going get him to go to school and like it (yeah right). I started to complain to the third teacher. I told her that I had dropped him off at school the previous Monday. I watched him come out the door at the end of the school day, but just found out that he had missed two periods that day. She reminded me that I was taking his responsibility away from him. I understood what she was telling me. Co-dependent behavior had sneaked up and caught me by surprise.

She gave me good advice. And few teachers would have taken the time to give that type of advice. My son's teacher was right. He needed to take responsibility for getting himself up and to the bus in the morning. I gave him that responsibility and consequently he dropped out of school. It will be his decision to reenroll when he is ready. I might be concerned that he will regret his decision one day, but he needs to be the one to experience the consequence of his decisions.

**2. Using Manipulation**

I've used manipulation throughout my life without realizing it. My decision to let my husband stay home to take care of our son was not a bad decision. I'm thankful that we were able to have one of us at home. At the time Joe was the best choice (he is far more domestic than I am). The unhealthy part of the decision was my reason for making it. I thought by keeping him without a means to earn money, I could keep him from abusing substances.

But my husband was very creative, he found ways to charge alcohol or trade for marijuana. As I paid huge bar bills, I suffered more, and he suffered less.

Our non-traditional decision to reverse the roles also created more stress because it was difficult for others to accept. It was through the use of manipulation that I thought I gained more control.

**3. Using control**

We have total control of our own life and none over those around us. In our practice of trying to control those around us, we give up the ability to control our own life. If our focus is aimed at the lives of others, we focus less on ourselves.

Controlling everything around me became so second nature that I didn't realize just how much I had to be in control. One of my first real breakthroughs regarding control was at work. Every time the department went out for lunch, I insisted on picking the restaurant. One time, another employee wanted to pick. I remember feeling a little competition because the other employee was not backing down. I finally gave over and allowed him to make the selection and guess what happened? The relief I felt was liberating. I started to wonder why I had not realized the responsibility that accompanied that little piece of control. When I took the responsibility of selecting the restaurant, I also took responsibility for whether the diners liked their lunch. This experience might sound insignificant, but it is through this type of awareness that I started to find I could safely let go of control and experience the release. And what a release it is!

(Controlling others can be a covert practice. Many times we don't even realize what we are doing.)

Our culture teaches being in control to us. Our parents do it to us with the most commendable of intentions, in the name of love. They do what they were taught, what their parents had done to them. They do it to smooth out our life path. They don't want us to have to experience unpleasantness. We learn this behavior from our parents and continue to use it with our children.

But no one has control of the lives of others. Each of us has to learn the lessons that we are destined to learn. We are on this earth to learn and grow, and it is through experiences, pleasant or unpleasant, that we do so. If, as parents, we try to take the unpleasantness out of the lives of our children, we are only prolonging the inevitable. When the lesson comes back to our child later in life, we might not be there with the needed support. Our child might not be emotionally strong enough to learn the lesson easily, because we have always been there to take their responsibility.

I followed our culture's standard when I became a parent. When my daughter was about six-years-old, I started to feel as though I was losing control over her. The truth was, I had already lost control. My daughter had learned how to gain control from a good teacher, me. She was calling the shots now and this made me uneasy, so I took her to a counselor. My complaint to Penny, our counselor, was that I couldn't get my daughter to do anything that I wanted her to do. Penny never did come out and say that it was my behavior that had caused the problem. She was smart enough to know that I would have reacted defensively.

Over the next three months, my daughter and I met with Penny separately. Penny conducted her session with my daughter while going to and from the store to purchase ice-cream cones. Penny and I met at the counseling center where she asked me to describe my experiences. I told her that my daughter would not get dressed, nor eat her breakfast in the morning. Each morning I could count on a battle, and unfortunately, my daughter seemed to be emerging, the victor. She would lackadaisically sit in front of her oatmeal. She seemed to think she had all day. In between getting dressed and putting on make-up, I would pick out what she would wear. I would say a silent prayer that she would feel okay about my selection and get dressed without a fight. Inevitably, I would end up helping her put on her shoes and socks minutes before we were to walk out the door. At the sitter's house, I would let a calm child out of the car. She didn't seem to have a care in the world. I, on the other hand, was thankful for the fifteen-mile commute that would give me time to unwind before I had to start work. I asked Penny to fix my daughter's stubborn behavior because it was causing way too much stress!

Penny asked what would happen if I let my daughter leave the house in her Pajamas without breakfast. I found myself describing how embarrassed I would feel bringing a child to the baby-sitter without breakfast in her PJs. What would the sitter think? Penny reminded me that it really didn't matter what the sitter thought. She went on to explain that my daughter would soon learn from her own embarrassment and hunger pains, and would make her own decision to get dressed and eat.

But then I would have to give up wanting my daughter to look a certain way. I had spent hours sewing little dresses and picking out matching accessories. I had ribbons for her hair and we spent many hours making sure that every hair was in place. Again Penny reminded me that my daughter needed to be the one to make the decisions regarding her appearance. Penny told me that even if she went to school with mismatched clothes, she needed to be the one to make the decision. As you can imagine, once I let go of trying to be in control, things changed considerably. My daughter went to the sitter in her pajamas without breakfast one time. She did not like missing breakfast, nor did she like being at the sitter's in her pajamas.

I tell my daughter today that her upbringing included dysfunctional behavior. I remind her that now she needs to get whatever help she needs to heal. There is no room for guilt or blame here. The past cannot be changed, but what we do with our experience can be.

After reading the story above, you can see just how easy it is to take someone's decision-making power away from him or her, in the name of "good parenting." Seeing a child immaculately dressed with their hair neatly arranged does not mean that that child is experiencing a healthy upbringing. Perfectionism is dysfunctional behavior, too.

When we deal with our loved ones, we need to ask ourselves why we select particular actions. Are we using our family to make ourselves look and feel better, as I did with my daughter? Is our perception of what is expected by society causing us to fear Judgement? Remember that we are in control over our perception of the societal rules, and we have the power to change our perception (more about how to change perception can be found in Chapter 7).

Think about how we feel when someone tries to control us by telling us what to do. Our first reaction is probably rebellion. Our loved ones are no different. Our loved ones are individuals, separate beings with their own needs and desires.

**4. Attaching**

When someone is attached, they will be adversely affected emotionally or economically by the decisions of the person they are attached to. Parents can become attached to children, and married people can become attached to one another. The family counselor at the Recovery Center illustrated the concept of attachment by drawing individual circles on the board representing family members. She drew two circles hooked together to illustrate an unhealthy attached relationship.

I practiced attachment unknowingly, because I didn't understand what being attached meant. My substance-addict's decisions were affecting me adversely, but I didn't realize that I was the one practicing unhealthy behavior. I believed that it was my substance-addict who had the problem, I was only trying to take care of my family's needs.

Our culture encourages some form of attachment between parents and children. In our society, parents are responsible for their children and will be held accountable for the child's wrongdoing if the child is under age. This implies that the parent is the only influence in the child's life and has in some way contributed to the wrongdoing of the child, and so deserves to be held responsible as well. Unfortunately the policy makers have taken the unfavorable consequence off the child and placed it on the parent.

I've been a parent to teen-agers two times, and I tend to disagree with this societal standard. If I try to force my teen to conform, I only seem to make matters worse. Detaching from our teens can also cause some more traditional members of our culture discomfort. But without detachment our teens will not feel some of the consequences of life, rather, we will.

As mentioned earlier, we as parents are obligated to give our children security, warmth, nurturance and guidance. There is a difference between guidance and trying to force our beliefs onto our child. We can share our beliefs, the rules and the consequences. We can follow through with enforcing the consequences, or allow our child to experience the consequences outside our control. I have found four important parental practices. They are not practices aimed at raising the perfect child. They are practices intended to support parental health:

- **I must show love to myself.**

If I want my children to have high self-esteem, I must have it myself.

- **I must strive to live my life the way I want my children to live theirs.**

Example is the best teacher.

- **I need to love my children unconditionally, whether or not they follow my rules or societal standards.**
- **I need to be aware of the traps of guilt and blame my children, or I might try to impose.**

If I take the blame, I take away my child's responsibility. It's important that I help them to understand that I have only done what I knew to do. If they are healthy enough to define a problem, they need to look for ways to find the healing.

Attachment to a child is more acceptable in our society than attachment to an adult. Becoming attached to a substance-addict is usually a part of the co-dependent/substance-addict experience. It's what brought the two players together. The substance-addict needed someone to take care of his or her needs. And the friend or family member needed someone to take care of. Taking care of the needs of others helps us feel whole.

I let go of attachment unknowingly a little at a time.

My detachment was done for survival. My husband and I owned one car for fifteen years of our marriage. I would drive it to work in the morning, and he would drive it to the bars at night. Many times I would find an empty gas tank when I got in it in the morning to go to work, which meant I usually had to be the one to fill it up with gas. This caused two problems: 1) we didn't have enough money to buy gas for trips to the bar, and 2) many mornings I was late because I didn't count on having to stop for gas (I should have figured that one out after a couple of gas pump stops). One morning I even ran out of gas on the way to the filling station!

After several months and many fueling stops, I looked for a way to cut costs. I found the answer in a carpool. I still had the refueling problem, but I only had to worry about it two weeks out of the month. Unfortunately carpooling created a new problem. My substance-addict could use the car on the days that I rode with my carpool. On these days he was expected to pick me up at the home of my carpool, and many times he didn't show up. I had to walk home and it was about three miles, in heels. My carpooling ended when my carpool partner moved. I started to ride the bus. Unknowingly, I had taken a giant step toward detachment. My husband had the car all of the time, but he had to be responsible for the gas. I had a reliable ride to and from work. I met some great people on the bus, and I spent the ride time, socializing, reading, listening to tapes or sleeping. It was liberating.

One late night my husband came into the bedroom. He woke me up and announced that the car had caught fire and was probably destroyed. Guess what? I didn't care. I had no emotion regarding the incident. I knew the insurance company would pay for the damage. The car was destroyed. I didn't even replace the car until I had to, three months later when we moved to Washington.

We can start to notice areas of attachment by analyzing our uncomfortable experiences. Are we feeling discomfort because of the actions of someone else? Are we the ones experiencing the consequences of their actions? Once we identify where we are attached, we can take small steps to detach.

**5. Enabling another to participate in unhealthy activity.**

It's easy to see how someone can become an enabler. When we are deeply attached to a substance-addict, we need to become an enabler to protect the entire family from going down. Again, I practiced enabling unknowingly. However, I was one of the best. Enabling is very covert and looks like the right thing to do, especially to those around us. I was just taking care of my family and making it work.

Enabling happens when we take away the responsibilities of the alcoholic, so that he/she never has to experience the repercussions. Rather we (family included) experience the repercussions for him/her.

Five years into our marriage, after trying control, manipulation, resentment, blame and self-pity with no luck, I moved my family one thousand miles away to Sumas, Washington. At the time, I didn't realize that my motivation to move was based on the belief that if I could get my substance-addict away from the problem, (his alcoholic friends) my problems would be solved. Before we left, he made a show of good faith by breaking his ceramic bong (a devise used to smoke marijuana). Are you laughing yet?

You know exactly what happened once we were established in our new location. My substance-addict met new friends that drank and drugged. He found a grocery store that would let him charge beer, and we continued in our new location right where we left off. This time though, I was one thousand miles away from my friends and family. We had few friends in the small community of Sumas. It was steeped in traditional religious beliefs. We did not live according to their religious teachings, and I felt they used alienation to deal with our disobedience.

My substance-addict didn't have to take responsibility for his actions because, according to me, his friends were at fault. I went so far as to tell my husband's best friend off for buying him alcohol for a Christmas present. My husband spent Christmas day passed out on the basement floor, and I blamed his friend. Now they both could understand the reason why he had to drink. With such a witch around, who could blame him?

In addition to the term "co-dependent", used to define dysfunctional behavior, there is the easier-to-take phrase "too much." It's a bit easier to be accused of doing "too much" because we are a culture that promotes overachievers.

Are we overachieving to keep from looking within? Or are we overachieving to fulfill a need? Are our needs healthy? If we are busy all the time, no one can accuse us of being a bad person.

Analyzing the underlying reason that we overachieve could help us understand and release any needs that might be unhealthy. Is our need based on the external? Are we concerned about what others think? Do we have to fit in with those around us? Do we care what the neighbors think? If we are overachieving to fulfill an external need, we must remember that we can only find lasting joy by feeling good about ourselves first. When we care too much about what others think, that is a signal that we are not accepting ourselves first. Once we start to feel good about ourselves first, we do not care what others think. I like the AA saying, "It's none of my business what others think of me." It's a good one to check to see if we are striving to find joy from external means.

Some other needs for overachieving: 1) taking on too much, so we can complain, 2) playing the victim, 3) volunteering, so we can be in control of the situation and those around us, 4) putting ourselves in uncomfortable situations as a form of punishment. Been there, done that.

The dysfunction I practiced had become so comfortable that it took me several years to realize that I avoided giving it up to get healthy. Many of my decisions were made in an attempt to control those around me. The longer I concentrated on controlling the external things in my life, the longer I could avoid looking inside. My feelings were strangers, and I was content to keep them that way.

I had become accustomed to the dysfunction around me. I was thankful that I had little time to spend with me. But discovering myself was an essential part of being human. If we don't or can't love ourselves, we have no feasible way to love others. We will turn away any love coming to us because, according to us, we are unlovable. If you are anything like me, looking in the mirror and saying, "I love you," is a hard thing to start doing.

The unhealthy practice of enabling, attachment, control and manipulation can be performed without full understanding. The individual can covertly practice these behaviors for many years with no way to pinpoint the dysfunction. In the years preceding my marriage to Joe, I saw a family counselor weekly for over six years. At the time I was a single parent struggling to maintain some degree of mental health. Each week my counselor listened to the sordid details of my life as I experienced one failed relationship after another, with one alcoholic after another.

I don't remember the counselor ever putting a finger on the dysfunction recognized as those associated with the friends and family members of substance-addicted individuals. Or, could it be that he did try to tell me, and I was so deep into toxic behavior that I didn't understand him? The best he could offer for treatment was for me to sit there and be listened to then go home and come back next week to start over. I'm not putting down that experience, but if this toxic behavior is so obvious and easy to spot and heal, then why didn't he notice, and help me to recover. One reason could be that research of the disease of substance abuse is still in its infancy. Consequently, information regarding the effects of the disease on the family is far from being fully understood.

With the proper diagnosis, could he have helped me to change my toxic behavior? Again, I have no judgement of the experience; it was a part of the life that created the person I am today.

We've identified unhealthy behavior practiced by me for many years. When the counselor at the Recovery Center told me to take my children and run, I somehow knew in my heart that leaving my husband wasn't the answer for me. If you are the spouse of an addict, divorce might be the answer for you. Only you can make that decision.

We can make our best decisions when we feel love and compassion for ourselves first. Becoming aware and taking responsibility, without blame are steps necessary on our path to self-love.

On our path we might find unhealthy behaviors such as judgement of ourselves. Harsh judgement of ourselves can cause us to become a victim. Our culture celebrates victims. We can watch the value of being a victim on television. Victims rake in the money from lawsuits, settlements, book or movie deals. We learn from example to dramatize the effects of uncomfortable experiences in our lives, and draw them out to the bitter end. I'm not saying that there aren't experiences in our lives that cause us pain and sorrow. But focusing on our negative experiences will not give us the opportunity to find our lesson and grow from the experience.

Keep in mind, we can be using victim-hood as a form of manipulation and control. I know because I've used being both a victim and a martyr. I used "going without", so that I could complain about it later, if I needed to. Being a martyr is unattractive. It doesn't take long for a family to 'get our number' when we play any game. Our family can turn around and play it back to us, by allowing us to go without, so there is more for them.

When one family member is playing victim or martyr, the entire group is out of sync. We learn best by experience. All of the covert game playing is noticed and being learned by our family members, especially the little ones. This is another good reason, for us to take care of ourselves first. Living the life we desire our family to live is the best gift we can give them. If we get ourselves on track first, it might throw the family off the dysfunctional balance they are used to, but they will respect us for it later.

Life is short. Experience the best life you can, your painful experience is a tiny drop in the bucket of eternity.

# Chapter 7

## Remember the Plan, Change Perception

*There appears to be physical limitations, yet experiences happen to individuals every day that fall outside our known physical limitation.*

It is easier for us to make inner permanent changes if we can believe that there is "a plan." At birth, we had to believe in "a plan." We were powerless. Something larger than ourselves created our existence. When we know that there is a Higher Power, we can go a step further and believe that there is "a plan". If we believe in "a plan", we can start to feel peace in our lives. With “a plan” belief, every event has a valuable purpose.

To believe in “a plan”, we will have to stretch our imagination and believe that there is more to life than what we feel, taste, see, hear and smell. Many of us are still looking at life through our five senses, trusting only in what we can prove and disprove using physical data. As humans, we can only physically see what is material, and from that perspective we can see many limitations. It might seem overwhelming for us to believe that there is a grand plan that includes each of us separately, and all of us together, especially when we look at the seemingly limited physical world around us.

There appears to be physical limitations, yet experiences happen to individuals every day that fall outside our known physical limitation. The experience is very real to the person living it. Most of us have read or heard about someone who has had a life after death experience. Many of these individuals will attest to a grander plan for their life that includes returning to their physical body. Individuals who have had out of the body experiences will also testify to life after death. What they experience is similar to the life after death experience.

If we believe in life after death, then we must believe that there is more than our physical body. We might call this “more than physical” part of us Spirit, Soul or Higher Self. This unseen yet felt part of us has much greater knowledge of the big picture and is a participating member in the plan. In addition, this unseen part of us is not limited by the constraints of the physical. It knows that there is more than our five senses, because it is "the more." Go a step further and know that this Higher Self wants only the best for you and the whole of creation. There is "a plan" for each of us, and our Higher Self is helping to make it become real.

"A plan" concept includes our finding and experiencing love. That objective may seem simplistic, but love is our greatest accomplishment; it is the root of all goodness. We don't truly understand love if we haven't found love for ourselves first. Not loving ourselves is no one's fault; we have no one to blame. It's just a part of our learning experience.

If there is a grand plan to our existence, and we have something to do with that plan, then why would we choose the life that we are living? Many of us feel that we are in situations that are impossible for us to escape. On the other hand, some of us don't want to escape them, because the familiar pain feels good. Much of the pain we experience could be transformed if we simply changed our perception of the experience.

We can start to change our perception by realizing that the events (even the painful ones) in our lives are there for our benefit. Each one of us is unique, with life experiences and beliefs that make our perception of life distinct. Consequently, your unique healing can't come from an outside source (me). It must come from the inside. I can only try to help you uncover the potential that lies within you.

Since healing and recovery is an inside job, a specific list of 'do and don't' suggestions for dealing with our substance-addict won't be in this book. This book was written to aid us in our inner recovery and healing, not how to react to our substance-addict. No one can tell us how to react to a specific situation, since each of us is unique with experiences and beliefs that are specific to us. Reactions need to come from a healed and recovered heart.

There is even a scripture that testifies to the availability of goodness (peace, joy and happiness) to all of us. A portion of Romans 8:28 states, "all things work together for *good*, for those who love the Lord". Many people perceive the scripture as saying that if we love the lord, all things good will happen to us.

Most of us have had experiences we perceived as uncomfortable. Thus, we wouldn't consider all things that happen to us as *good*. If we do believe in a Higher Power, we could put ourselves on quite a guilt trip when we interpret the scripture to mean that the discomfort will be removed from our lives if we love the Lord. We can choose to perceive the scripture as saying that **all things work together** for *good*. If all things do work together for *good*, we can see each experience we have as a fragment of a much larger picture. We may have initially defined some of our experiences as *bad,* but in a larger picture we can see that they eventually work together for the benefit of all. In some cases, we may never see the benefit to someone we met briefly. Our *bad* experience may have been a positive life-changing event for another individual, without our knowledge.

If we look back over our life, we might discover an experience that we perceived as *bad* then realized later its place as a valued part of the larger picture. I have a good example of this principle.

About twenty-two years ago, I was fired from my job as a claims representative for an automobile insurance company. To me, that was an ultimate *bad* thing. I was a single parent with the responsibility of supporting my daughter and myself. What would I do without a job? I went to the unemployment office to apply for unemployment. At the unemployment office, I was sobbing so profusely that I could barely fill out the paperwork.

My perception at the time was that only irresponsible people were fired from their jobs. What a guilt trip! Now, I look back on that experience, and I am thankful that I was fired from that job. As a claims representative, I had to deal with people who had been involved in automobile accidents. Occasionally, I didn't agree with the decision of upper management regarding claim payments. In addition, it was difficult for me to ask a bereaved relative where they took the body. The job was not right for me, yet I never would have quit, since I was trying to maintain my perception of a responsible adult. A responsible adult worked to earn a living whether they liked the job they were doing or not. To me, work wasn't something you enjoyed. That's why they called it work. Of course, I found a much better job after being fired that supported my family for twenty-two years. Even though that job had its ups and downs, in the larger picture I can say that

I learned many valuable life lessons from it. And those lessons will serve me for many years.

It's the uncomfortable experiences that teach us the most valuable lessons. We can change our perception of rules; and rather than wallow in the discomfort, we can choose to see all of our experiences as adventures.

I've often wondered where societal rules came from, and who determined what they would be in the first place. In a society made up of so many different types of individuals, it seems that some rules would become obsolete as the world grows in diversity. We also have rules we were taught as youngsters by our parents, teachers, religious leaders and peers. It could also be that some of our individual rules are no longer working for us.

As we become aware and take responsibility, we should reevaluate our rules. It might be time to change the way we perceive them. Or even delete some of the ones that don't work for us now that we have become adults. Once we reevaluate our rules, we might find that we could let up on the judgement and the consequences of breaking the rules. We end up light-hearted and relieved, making us go a little easier on our loved ones and ourselves.

Our rules had to come from the comparisons of one person's behaviors to the behaviors of another person: how the majority of individuals act in a situation, and what consequences are experienced. With these comparisons, we are still using the external to measure how we are doing. Again, it is only the inside that we can change. Inside, we can change the way we perceive the rules. Once we release ourselves from the high expectations of these rules, detachment and acceptance become much easier. One can find relief in the spiritual belief that there is a larger plan (and that belief sometimes comes over time) where all things work together for good.

When I tell people of my experiences, I get mixed reactions. Some bring up their own definitions of the societal rules. Some dislike my husband for being an alcoholic, while others think I'm an idiot for staying with him, and some people think I'm a saint. But in the eyes of most, my behavior was acceptable; I was the good guy. I was following the rules of being a good wife. But I was taking care of matters using control and manipulation. Because of these misunderstandings, my part in the toxic behavior continued unrecognized for years.

I was following the rules, but in a dysfunctional way. Healing won't begin while we are being praised for our behavior. It's when our lives become chaotic that we seek help and understanding. As friends and family members of substance-addicts, our lives start to become unmanageable when we try to maintain some type of regular life with a person who has changed the rules. Substance-addicts have exchanged human nurturance for a substance. And that substance becomes far more important to them than the human nurturance.

In the same way we change our perceptions of *good* and *bad* experiences we can change our perception of *good* and *bad* individuals. Stuart Wilde, in his book entitled *Infinite Self,* states,

> *"All negative energy comes from the perceptions and definitions of the ego. What we call misfortune, or negative experience, is any contradiction of the ego's opinion."*

Wilde's statement suggests that we define good and bad experiences based on a deep-rooted belief or definition of self. That definition is developed from our experiences and the beliefs taught to us by our parents and society. Those beliefs become our measuring stick. We make judgements of ourselves, our experiences and those around us by comparing what we see to our perception of how life should be. When we re-define our beliefs, first our perceptions and then our experience begins to change.

Perceptions vary from country to country. There is a delightful member of my Toastmaster's group who moved to the United States from China a few years ago. Her perceptions are much different than ours, yet we cannot consider them as either right or wrong. One week she chose the word *destiny* as our word of the day, because it was a word without meaning in her country. Each individual born in China is predestined, based on factors such as the time of birth and the physical appearance. This concept seemed funny to the audience. I imagine our traditional beliefs seem a bit silly to her and the people from her country. The fact that the many individuals from China believe these factors to determine the future of its citizens makes that belief a reality.

We can change our perceptions by becoming aware of our impulsive judgements. We can ask ourselves where our measuring stick came from. Just because it's right for us, doesn't mean it's right for others, as with my example of my friend from China. We can start to ask ourselves what beliefs we learned as a child, from a parent, a sibling, a friend or a religion that has caused us to make a judgement. Is the judgement valid? Is it necessary? Any negative judgement we have can be dissolved, or neutralized if we stop and find out what belief we have that has caused us to feel the way we do. We can ask ourselves again whether our belief is still valid for us.

Once we change our perceptions, we can reap the benefits of inner peace that come with non-judgement of self and others. It is easier to love one another when there are no unrealistic expectations. We can start small, redefine some beliefs and discover the seed that planted that negative judgement, then purge it from the garden of our heart. We can nurture the seeds of love and start to see the goodness inside and outside of ourselves.

Again, perceptions we have that cause us to make judgements of others and ourselves can be lessened if we believe that there is an ultimate plan. With "a plan" concept we can accept without judgement that everyone is where he or she needs to be. Each of us can and will find within our hearts the belief that offers us the best opportunity to experience love. Whether it is through "a plan" concept or through more traditional religious teachings. Many of us, myself included, have been taught that this life is a test, and that there are many of us humans who fail the test. In the concept of "a plan" there is no test, but only life experiences to be learned, for the benefit of the whole of creation.

I changed my belief from a life-test belief to a belief, which includes an all-powerful non-judgmental loving Creator. Our Creator brings the sun and the rain. The rain is often judged to be the more unpleasant of the two, yet it takes both sun and rain for Mother Nature and her children to survive. In the same way, it takes both comfortable and uncomfortable experiences, for us to become whole beings.

The opposite of "a plan" belief, the life-test belief includes a judgmental God who emerges with conditional love for creation. If a part of creation commits sin throughout the life-test experience, it will be cast away from God for eternity. The book used as the reference for this belief, the *Bible*, maintains that it is God's desire to save all men. Logically, if God is "The All That Is" then he can have what he desires. God makes his power known in the *Bible* when he says through his prophets, "my will be done."

In "a plan" belief, you are reading this book because there is beneficial information in it for you, whether you agree with all of its contents or not.

The "plan" belief that includes an unconditional god becomes easier to accept if we are willing to consider reincarnation. With the concept of reincarnation, we have the opportunity to have many earth-plane experiences. For further understanding, reincarnation can be compared to our current life experience. By the time we reach adulthood, we have been an infant, an adolescent, a young adult and an adult. All of these phases have worked together to make us who we are in this lifetime. In the same way, our many life incarnations make up our Higher Self. With the reincarnation belief, we can choose each visit back to earth, based on our other life experiences. If we experienced being a slave owner in one life, we may choose to experience the life of a slave in the next, for balance.

Whether we believe in "a plan" concept or not, we can change our perception of how others should behave. We can choose to relinquish our seat in the courtroom as judge and jury. We can start to see the goodness in others and accept them for who they are. If we see judgement rather than goodness, we can ask ourselves why we have that judgement. Sometimes that judgement is our Higher Power showing us something we need to work on.

For many years I didn't believe in "a plan" concept. Rather, I rebelled against the perceived judgement of an enemy: society. As a single parent in 1973, I believed that I was being judged by society because I was a single parent. At the time I didn't realize that it was my own belief and judgement creating the discord I was experiencing. I was making judgements of my actions based on my perceived societal rules. Rather than just change my definition of what was acceptable for me, I rebelled. I lived with an, "I'll show them," attitude. I had the belief that God was available, but that he was allowing my life to be uncomfortable as a form of punishment. Now I can see that that is a silly notion. I was struggling against my own beliefs and judgements, then blaming God and society for their staunch rules.

Now I believe that there is “a plan”, I do not judge my actions because I believe my experiences have been just as they needed to be. That includes <u>all</u> of my past experiences. My experiences have led to this place of realization.

Our own perception of ourselves is very powerful and can influence others. The following story is embarrassing for me, but it has such a powerful message, I must tell it. I met a woman some time ago whose nose seemed a bit long. However, she accepted the face she had been given. Her positive energy was so apparent that it wasn’t long before her belief became mine. I soon realized that her nose wasn’t long, in fact it worked together with her face to make her a very beautiful woman. That’s how powerful our own beliefs can be! Our perceptions of ourselves affect the beliefs of those around us. I’m thankful to my friend, for that powerful lesson in self-acceptance and non-judgement.

We can change our perception of others when we understand what motivates them. We can understand what motivates them by recognizing their differences. I learned this great lesson regarding our differences at the ropes-course seminar I mentioned earlier. At one time during the seminar we broke into small groups of about six. Each one of us got six minutes to share our differences. As each person shared their differences, preconceived beliefs about that person evaporated. A clearer understanding of the motivations of each person in that room emerged. Before we pass judgement on others we can consider their differences.

We can celebrate our differences. They are what make us the unique human beings we are today. During a time of self-doubt (self-doubt can sneak up on us, the good news is, it doesn't last), I called my friend Jackie in Washington to share my fears about writing this book.

I asked her if she thought I was wasting my time. "What if there are other books just like it?"

She said, "If you have two blue puzzle pieces, do you throw one away? No, it takes all of the blue puzzle pieces to make up the sky in the puzzle." (I have some wise friends. Don't I?)

In the same way that it takes all of the blue puzzle pieces, it takes each one of us as unique individuals to make up the whole of creation!

Understanding our differences will help us to accept ourselves with love and compassion. The acceptance of ourselves will influence acceptance by those around us.

We change our negative thoughts to positive thoughts about ourselves and change our lives. We change our negative thoughts to positive thoughts about those around us and change their lives. When we are focusing on the positive qualities of others, we react to them differently. All too often, we focus on the negative actions of others to justify our own feelings. Instead, we can try looking for the positive actions of that person. We can find a few things that we really like about them. We can go a step further, and tell them what qualities we've noticed.

When we catch ourselves perceiving others in a negative way, we need to ask why we feel the way we do. Everything outside of us is a reflection to teach us more about our own self.

When we get to the place in life where we become aware, take responsibility and trust the Universe completely to supply us with all we need to exist and fulfill our purpose in this lifetime we do not need to employ dishonesty. I'm not making a judgement of dishonesty I'm only trying to show how it can send a powerful message that can limit our possibilities. When we practice dishonesty, we are attempting to manipulate the outcome. When we try to manipulate the outcome, we are defining the outcome <u>we</u> think is best. We as humans have a limited view of the possibilities, whereas the Universe is comprised of millions of possibilities and probabilities. Why would we want to use our limited view to manipulate an outcome when the universal possibilities are limitless? Why are we trying to control and mold the future to secure the outcome we think is best? Our defined outcome may not be the best for all concerned. We are setting ourselves up for possible disappointment and self-judgement if our desired outcome doesn't "pan-out" as we had expected.

Sometimes we feel as though we can justify our dishonesty in our financial endeavors. We might decide to practice dishonesty on our income tax return to avoid paying large sums of money to the government. We might justify our actions with the belief that the government has enough of our money, or that they don't make good use of the money they have. Not only are we breaking the earthly law with this action, we are sending a powerful message to the Universe and ourselves. The message we send is that we don't believe we have the ability to earn enough money without using dishonesty. We are putting a limitation on the amount of money we believe we can earn.

We can attempt to be honest with ourselves regarding our actions. We can get to the core of our choices by asking, what are our motivations? Are we trying to manipulate a desired outcome? We always need to remember to become aware and take responsibility without judgement. Our past actions are not brought to light, so that we can inflict punishment. If we find toxic behavior, we can simply purge it, thank the Universe for the awareness, forgive ourselves for any perceived indiscretion, defuse any disabling beliefs and move on.

Guilt is what we feel when we think we could have done something different to get a different result. Once we embrace the concept of "a plan," both guilt and shame (the act of judging ourselves as bad) become emotions of the past.

We've discussed the fact that we have no control over others, that we are only responsible for ourselves.

We've talked about a grand plan orchestrated to help us to learn and to love. We've discovered that some of our best learning comes through uncomfortable experiences. If all of this is true, then there should be no guilt or shame.

Guilt is a by-product of judgement. In a world where all things work together for good, there should be no judgement. We might feel guilt because we have set standards we expect others to comply with, then we find ourselves not complying. We have no right to expect others to fit our expectations, because everyone's experience makes them unique. There is no "one standard fits all".

There are no "should haves" or "could haves" in a life that is being lived according to "a plan". We may ask, "How do I know I'm living according to the plan?" It is because our Higher Self and the Universe are assisting us to insure we accomplish the adventures and lessons we are here to experience.

Feeling guilty should be a clue to us to look at some perceptions about what we believe should have been. Our "should have been" might be based on beliefs that no longer work for us. If we are experiencing discomfort because of guilt, we have the power to dissolve that discomfort.

In the same way that our Higher Self and the Universe are working together for our higher good, our loved ones are working with their Higher Self and the Universe. Non-judgement and acceptance will fill our life with peace, joy and happiness.

When we choose non-judgement, we accept the circumstances that happen in our life, and the lives of those around us. Consequently, there is no guilt or shame. Peace is obtainable when we see the value of those circumstances as necessary happenings occurring to aid in the growth of all individuals involved. There is an overall plan being orchestrated by our Creator. Our Creator knows exactly what circumstances we all need to experience to fulfill our purpose in this lifetime. When we make a negative judgement of ourselves, we are sending a powerful message that we are lacking, incomplete or defective. With that negative judgement, we create a belief that will season our future life experiences. Not only will we affect our own life with the negative judgement; we will project it out to those around us.

Each of us is a unique individual on our own life path. If we make a negative judgement of a certain action we might deny ourselves our greatest life lesson. Or when we are acting in harmony with our Higher Power, we can choose to lighten up on judgement and trust that all things work together for good.

If we can learn to practice forgiveness, we can start to dissolve guilt and shame. Earlier, I wrote that we feel guilt and shame because we are judging an action that we have taken as not being right. When we make judgements, we are not trusting in the ability of our Creator to select the adventures that are in our greatest interest. Once we have trust in the Creator to bring about the valuable lessons associated with all experience, we can forgive those around us and ourselves. If we find it difficult to forgive, we must go within and ask our Higher Power what lessons we need to learn. Again, everything outside of us is a reflection of ourselves. If we don't like what we see outside, we can go inside to find out why. Judgements start inside of us. We had to experience it within ourselves first before we could identify in someone else. Unresolved resentments based on judgements will continue to draw reflections in the outside world like a magnet. Our Higher Power will continue to bring individuals or experiences into our life to help us see where we need improvement until we "get the picture".

In addition, we give our energy away to those we cannot forgive. Those unpardonable sins consume our time and take up valuable space in our mind, space that could be used for our own enlightenment. In AA, there is a saying, "Don't let someone take up space in your mind rent-free."

Throughout my life I've made negative judgements of many of my life experiences. Specifically, I still needed to work on judgement, for doing something I considered "bad" and guilt and regret for breaking the perceived societal rules. Stuffing these toxic judgements may cause beliefs of unworthiness later. When we don't feel worthy, we stop ourselves from receiving the gracious gifts from the Universe.

To dissolve these judgements, I used my imagination to gather my perceived indiscretions and load them on a bus. Many of my judgements involved other individuals. I watched the group visit amongst themselves as they waited to board the bus.

Occasionally, one would turn around and wave at my guide and me. I smiled and waved back feeling no regret. They loaded on the bus and it drove off. Some leaned out the window and waved good-bye. I waved too and was glad to see them get on their way and out of my belief system. I both accepted them, and let them go using my imagination. Our imagination helped us to find self-hate. Let it help us find self-love. We can give ourselves the gift of self-love. It might be hard for us to love ourselves if we harbor regret.

Every experience we have is one more step toward our purpose in this life. If we regret something from our past, we are saying that things could have or should have worked out differently. When we look back over our lives, we can find how the experiences we might now regret have caused other events to happen which positively effected our lives or the lives of others. Every experience has happened in our lives to create the individuals that we are today. If we don't like what we see, remember that we are still in the process of creation. If we look at life through non-judgmental eyes, one day we will get the opportunity to see how each and every experience fits neatly into a much larger and more important plan. We can start to see our regrets as new adventures that will take us down a path we hadn't expected. We may be affecting people in a way that isn't obvious to us at this time and may never be.

Ten years ago I didn't know that one day I would take the pain I was feeling, and use it to reach out to others experiencing the same pain. Ten years ago it was hard to see how I could even make it through each day. Life was so painful that I asked to stay another day in the hospital after surgery in 1988. I didn't want to go home to the dysfunction there. Some of the seemingly most insignificant experiences of my life are now showing up to help with what I believe to be my life's purpose. I worked in the graphics department of my company when I moved back from Washington. At the time, it would not have been my choice because the challenge of the position was less than I had been used to. I realize now that it was a good place, to start my healing process. Now that I'm working on self-publishing this book, I can see how invaluable that graphic experience was for me. I have a greater understanding of the printing process because I worked with printers and graphic designers.

When we believe in "a plan", it is easier to accept our past, to embrace it then release our regrets in non-judgement. The Universe has worked to get us to this point. It will continue to take us to the next step and the next. Learn to trust that there is a greater good to all of our life experiences.

We can start to release regret when we realize that we are human BEINGS, living only in the present. When we let past experiences consume our thoughts; we give away our energy. We should only venture into our past for the purpose of non-judgmental healing. Our future is our opportunity to experience adventure. But we need not be concerned about it, because it is our present that creates our future. Our present should be our only concern. We should be thankful, for the perfect order of the Universe, and our unique place in it. We need to accept that tomorrow may be uncomfortable, but with the discomfort there will be a tremendous learning opportunity. When we worry about the future, we send the signal that we are not happy with today. Rather, let's celebrate today and work on self-love by doing something special for us. Chocolate malts anyone?

# Chapter 8

## Self-Love...What's Keeping Us From It?

*The emergency room attendants did something that I should have done months earlier; they threw out that pair of ratty underwear.*

We can begin to discover self-love by changing our thoughts, our perceptions and our disabling beliefs. These few simple thought process changes will drastically change our lives.

We must love ourselves first. To some that might sound selfish. If we don't love ourselves first, we do not know the true definition of love. Without the true definition of love, we can't give it to anyone.

It must come from the inside. I can only try to help you uncover the self-love that lies within you. With a firm foundation of self-love the perception of events as painful will be lessened. When we have self-love, we have a foundation of confidence. With this confidence, those outside events no longer have the power to affect us. I hope that by sharing what I've learned about loving myself, I can help you to find the same peace, joy and happiness available to all of us.

If we look at how we treat ourselves, we might notice some unhealthy dishonoring behavior. We could be dishonoring ourselves by "going without" and not buying ourselves nice things. This action is a good indication that we don't believe we deserve to have nice things. Or we could be doing the opposite by going out and buying up everything in an effort to cover-up low self-esteem.

We could be dishonoring ourselves unknowingly as I was in the following example. I was in an automobile accident about twenty years ago. I don't know if my mother actually said to me, "always wear your best underwear, just in case you are in an accident," or if it was just a common belief. (If you are younger than I am, you might not have heard this advice. I certainly hope that mothers have stopped giving that fear-based advice.) The day of my accident I had on some of the rattiest underwear known to woman. You might have some like them: stretched out elastic, rips, faded color, the works. What I realize now, as I look back over the incident, is that continuing to wear that pair of underwear sent a powerful dishonoring signal to me.

(Mothers should be telling their children, "always wear your best underwear because you deserve the best.")

The emergency room attendants did something that I should have done months earlier; they threw out that pair of ratty underwear. By keeping and wearing them, I was sending a message to myself that I didn't deserve to have nice things.

It's a funny story, but I share it to drive home the point that we can unknowingly treat ourselves disrespectfully.

But buying ourselves new underwear isn't going to cause us to miraculously start to show respect and love to ourselves. We can be told that loving ourselves is the best gift we can give to our loved ones and to ourselves. But until we understand why we don't practice love for ourselves, the words are meaningless. We may not love ourselves because we are harboring some dishonoring beliefs about ourselves unknowingly. These beliefs could have grown from an off-the-wall comment said to us when we were young and impressionable. Unrecognized disabling beliefs can continue to affect how we experience life. They can even prevent us from experiencing peace and joy. I shared earlier that from life experiences as a youngster, I had believed for many years that I was unworthy, unlovable and not deserving.

In addition to believing that I was unworthy, unlovable and not deserving, I had a belief that I had committed sin and broken societal rules. Based on this belief, I had judgement of myself, and I feared the judgement of others. I held unrealistic expectations of myself based on my perception of sin and the rules of society. In truth, I alone had control over my definition of sin and rules (discussed in Chapter 7). I could have changed that perception and stopped the harsh internal judgement at any moment. I was my worst enemy. In reality, those perceived infractions contained some of my most valuable learning experiences. Once I realized that those internal judgements were preventing me from finding self-love, I could transmute them. Now I can give thanks, for my valuable life lessons without judgement or blame.

We must be careful not to blame others or ourselves or make judgements of the disabling beliefs we uncover. To judge our life thus far would be to start another disabling belief, the belief that we have done something wrong. Rather, we have not done something wrong, we have developed more opportunities for growth and expansion! Identifying those beliefs gives us the opportunity to thank God, for the lessons those beliefs have taught and will continue to teach us. They all offer great value. We can thank God that we have discovered them and ask for the strength to change them to beliefs that suit our current needs. We can remember the trust we had as a newborn and believe that there is "a plan" and that everything is as it should be. We can begin to accept whatever has happened in the past and whatever the future brings to those around us and ourselves. We can start to see our future and the future of our loved ones as an adventure. A future filled with the excitement and the potential for growth.

We can learn to trust and accept the gracious gifts of the Universe with a fuller understanding of our Higher Power.

Sometimes the belief was instilled with good intention, as was the following example that went unnoticed for many years.

While growing up, if I came to my mother with a complaint about another individual, she always asked me, "What did <u>you</u> do?" I understand now that she was trying to teach that disagreements usually take two. Recently I realized that I continually asked myself what I had done wrong each time there was a misunderstanding with someone else. Many times disagreements with others have nothing to do with what I did wrong, but rather are an issue with the other individual. Although my mother's advice was well meant, I had a disabling belief that I had to change.

Many experts believe that buried under disabling beliefs is a fragile inner child. This inner child is creative and pure. Julia Cameron wrote the book, *The Artist's Way,* and developed a course to help people recover that inner creative child. Julia wrote *The Artist's Way* after she started her alcohol addiction recovery. She was prompted to write the book because she feared that she would lose her creativity with her sobriety. She developed a twelve-week course to recover her inner creative child. She believed this inner creative child was hidden under layers of beliefs and myths.

My husband and I took *The Artist's Way* course. During the course, students are encouraged to participate in activities designed to awaken their inner creative child. As I participated in the weekly activities, I realized that the tasks encouraged self-nurturing. Many of them were activities we enjoyed as children, but activities we view as childish now that we are adults. The activities are designed to help us remember ourselves before we were stifled with the shoulds and should nots bestowed upon us by well-meaning individuals.

As I completed each week of activities, old belief patterns started to emerge. Our instructor, Rick Graham, used the classroom experience to help students identify some old patterns, beliefs and myths. Once we started to feel the freedom we experienced as children, we discovered the beliefs that kept us from feeling that freedom in our lives today. Julia's program is not only beneficial to those individuals, who believe they are artists, but for anyone who wants to find their inner creative child.

Becoming aware of disabling beliefs and then dissolving them is a good way to discover why we continue to do things that are not for our higher good. Some of our beliefs may have triggered our fragile inner child to develop a personality for protection. Hal and Sidra Stone have written several books on the psychology of multiple personalities (selves). The Stones believe that our inner child will create alter-personalities for protection. I am not referring to multiple personality disorder, used many times as a defense by criminals. Rather, individuals use these less prominent personalities unknowingly at times of perceived need. The Stones teach that some of the selves that our inner child has created no longer offer a positive experience for the adult we have become. The Stones have developed a procedure called, "voice dialogue" to help discover and understand the selves and their purpose.

Rick Graham, our instructor in *The Artist's Way* is a facilitator in the technique of voice dialogue.

Throughout the course, Rick facilitated voice dialogue sessions with a few of the students. During the voice dialogue session, Rick talks to the individual personalities that developed based on Hal and Sidra Stones' theory. I watched with interest as the participants allowed their other personalities to surface and talk with Rick. With prompting from Rick, they explain why they feel the need to be a part of the individual's life. Their reasons for developing seemed valid. For one student, the critical self had to develop because if not for it, the individual would be unable to accomplish anything meaningful in life.

On my way home from class one evening, I realized that I had what I will call my "financial self." This personality came into being out of a belief in the need for security when I became responsible for a family. My financial self has spent countless hours reviewing where the money would come from, and where it would go. My financial self spent time adding and re-adding, arranging and rearranging. The problem is that this behavior is practiced in the fear of lack, and we draw what we put our most emotional energy into. In addition, when my financial self is reviewing my money situation, limitations are being set on where money can come from and where money needs to go.

Some time ago, I realized that my disabling beliefs of being unworthy and not deserving were affecting my financial health. My beliefs had developed into a fear that I would never have enough money to cover expenses. I asked for help with my money issues from the Universe. Bit by bit, I have learned how to gain trust in the unconditional support of the Universe. I found that not only did I believe that I was unworthy and not deserving, but I believed that there was only a limited amount of money. These are serious disabling beliefs!

Many times we find it hard to discontinue our disabling beliefs and believe in something that is a spiritual truth if we continue to experience what we see as its opposite. Usually we are experiencing the opposite because of a hidden deep-rooted belief. To change our unpleasant experiences, we need to locate our disabling beliefs so that we can change them.

Disabling beliefs can prevent us from experiencing the idea expressed in the Bible scripture Matthew 6:26, which testifies that the Universe does desire to support us in our needs.

> *Behold the fowls of the air: for they sow not, neither do they reap, nor do they gather into barns; yet your heavenly Father feedeth them. Are ye not much better than they?*

That scripture gives me comfort. I hope it will do the same for you. We do have a loving and giving Universe. If I look back over my life experience, I can see that my beliefs were unfounded, because my needs have always been met. Unfortunately, my belief prevented me from enjoying more of the abundant gifts offered by our gracious Universe.

Even with the comforting scripture, I had some deep-rooted beliefs to transmute in order to stop my frightened financial self from figuring and re-figuring every cent. I decided there was only one thing I could do and that was to offer my financial self, early retirement. (Our imagination is a powerful tool.) I offered my financial self room and board and board and board, for the rest of her life. I suggested she spend her free time sitting on the beach, drinking marguerites. I thanked her for her years of service and acknowledged her contribution to our success. (After all, she is a financial genius! She has always been there to help make things work out, one way or another. Even if it was by robbing Peter to pay Paul). I told her that I had decided it was time to try another approach, and that approach was trust in the Universe. I offered her contract work if a time arises that I need her expertise again. She stays on the beach most of the time, if she does decide to mettle, I remind her of our deal and send her back.

The retirement of my financial self might sound silly and extreme to you, but I needed to change some very embedded beliefs. Why not have a little fun with it?

We've discussed how the selves are created from a belief, and at the time they are a much-needed support system. But as we grow, and our lives change, some of our beliefs and the selves created by them are no longer needed. Instead of providing the protection initially intended, the selves and the belief block our potential. Rick told us that we cannot completely rid ourselves of the selves, and when identifying them, it is important to acknowledge their contribution. However, I do believe we can change the belief that prompted their creation. For more information, read the many books regarding the selves written by Hal and Sidra Stone. Call a voice dialogue facilitator and schedule a session. Or use a technique called cognitive therapy.

At the Alcohol and Drug Treatment Training Program I am attending at the University of Utah, we learned about cognitive therapy in one of our classes. Cognitive therapy is an exercise used to recognize and stop inaccurate thinking. An event, called a trigger, will prompt thinking; the thinking can be negative and inaccurate. Negative feelings can follow the negative thinking, which can cause inappropriate behavior. Generally, negative consequences follow inappropriate behavior. Analyzing and changing the negative thinking following a trigger can prevent inappropriate behavior and the subsequent unpleasant consequences. The thinking following a trigger can be very personal negative beliefs that have nothing to do with the current situation. When they are analyzed rationally they can be changed to more realistic thinking.

I experienced the theory of cognitive thinking the same evening of the class on the subject. While our instructor was demonstrating the procedure with students, I raised my hand to share the concept of the selves and voice dialogue. The instructor called on me and I shared my thoughts. She told me that voice dialogue was a more involved process than she was teaching in this class. Her dismissal of my comment was a trigger for me. Very negative personal thoughts started to race through my mind, *she's read my book and she disagrees with it, my input is not valuable, I don't know what I'm talking about, I'm a looser.* The feelings that came from those thoughts were devastating. I felt worthless, sad and depressed. The behavior that followed was short-lived, but very real. I wanted to give up on my book, on my speaking and on my studies. I just wanted to drop out of life. All of this happened in about a 2-minute time frame. I realized that I had just experienced a trigger, which started negative thoughts, followed by negative feelings, prompting contemplation of negative behavior. You know as well as I, when my teacher told me she didn't want to go into voice dialogue, that's all she meant. Her comment was not directed at me personally. This is a simple example, one that most of us would not let go beyond contemplation of negative behavior. But I share it to show how easy it is to get from trigger to thoughts of negative behavior. In addition, the thinking prompted by the trigger can be very personal, and most likely inaccurate, as in my example. Again, thought is very powerful.

As we've discussed, thoughts can be utilized in a positive way, as in the example of my financial self's retirement. In the same way, I can think positively about myself to change my life. Positive thoughts can neutralize negative thoughts, and before long they can change lives. My first experience with this life-changing truth came in about 1982 after I read the book, *Psycho-cybernetics* by Maxwell Maltz, M.D., F.I.C.S.

Dr. Maltz suggests that our sub-conscious is a servomechanism, operating off data input by our thoughts with no judgement of that data. The data input can be positive or negative; our servomechanism acts equally on both. Dr. Maltz has many examples to prove this theory. Based on Dr. Maltz's theory, we would be much better off if we could give our servomechanism positive input.

I used my thoughts to put Dr. Maltz's theory to the test. At the time, I was from fifteen to twenty pounds overweight. I had tried most of the fad diets available. I was constantly thinking about my weight (and remember we draw what we put our emotional energy into). I was always on the verge of starting a new diet, so I would overeat the day before. Rather than have one donut I would have three. I feared that I might not get the chance to eat another donut ever again. I figured I had better get my fill when I could. In his book, Dr. Maltz suggests that we decide the weight we want to be then start to believe we are that weight. I selected my ideal weight and started to believe. A neat thing happened: I stopped wanting to overeat! I ate only when I was hungry and stopped when I was full (guilt for wasting food was another disabling belief I had to uncover and change). Today I am at my desired weight and have not dieted or been concerned about my eating habits since.

My experiment with thought proves what Dr. Wayne W. Dyer writes in his book *Real Magic*, that our thoughts create our experiences. Our thoughts are very powerful. If we look back over our life, we can see what we have created. If doctors Maltz and Dyer are correct, each time we say a negative thing about ourselves, our body responds. Our body accommodates our request by sending out the request and making it so.

I discuss the potential of positive thought in my booklet *Seven Ways to Positively Believe Yourself off the Diet Roller Coaster* by referencing the teachings of the two authors mentioned above. I try to convince my readers to stop saying and thinking that they are fat, that they need to lose pounds, or that they might as well glue the food they are about to eat onto their hips. All are very powerful words and thoughts that are self-destructive and give the dieter the opposite of what they really desire.

When we think negatively about ourselves, we create a pathway for it to come back to us from the outside world. If we want the self-destructive experiences to stop, we must stop the negative self-talk. If we start becoming aware of the negative talk that comes out of our mouth, or goes through our mind, we will be surprised. We need to stop announcing that we don't have enough money, that we are losing our mind (one I catch myself using), or that we are stupid. If we can stop this unhealthy behavior, we can simply change our negative experiences into positive experiences. Affirmations are so powerful!

We can start to change our negative thoughts by becoming aware. When a negative thought pops into our mind, we can change it to a positive thought. Dr. Dyer suggests that we don't use any part of the negative talk. An example would be instead of, "I am not losing my mind," rather "I am gaining my mind." It sounds silly, but it was that phrase I had to change.

Negative talk (derived from negative thought) is rampant. We hear it everywhere we go. My former boss had a great saying, "What comes out of your mouth goes into your life."

Go further with this concept, what past negative thoughts are causing negative experiences for you today? What positive thoughts can you create to mold the life you want tomorrow? This may sound simplistic, but there are examples of this belief based on scientific data, as in Multz's book, *Psycho-cybernetics* and the spiritual beliefs as in, Dr. Dyer's, book *Real Magic*.

When we talk positively to ourselves, we should look into the mirror and say, "I love you." Put emphasis on the word you, "I love you." Point at yourself as you say I, then point at your reflection when you say you, "I love you." Sing it, "I love you, yeah, yeah, yeah." Look deep into the reflection of your eyes and say, ***"I love you."***

Affirmations can help us to get to the place where we truly love ourselves at the core. With love for ourselves we can to start to experience peace, joy and happiness. It's time to stop avoiding ourselves and start identifying the feelings we have about ourselves.

As I discovered, beliefs about sin and punishment can prevent us from receiving answers to our prayers.

Affirmations are a great way to uncover some of those old, disabling beliefs. As we start to talk positively to ourselves, and yes I mean while looking into the mirror, those buried negative beliefs will pop into our minds. Julia Cameron in *The Artist's Way*, calls these blurts. She suggests writing them down to help discover where they came from, so that they can be changed into positive truths. In *Real Magic*, Dr. Dyer suggests saying affirmations whether we believe them or not. Louise L. Hay, writes in her book, *You Can Heal Your Life*, that looking into the mirror and saying positive things about us is a powerful tool. Louise points out that someone looking us directly in the eye gave much of the negative information we received as a child. We can reverse those messages by looking ourselves in the eye and saying positive things about ourselves. All the teachers who support affirmations encourage us to go beyond what we think is enough, to repeat positive messages to ourselves many times. Most of us probably have lots of negative beliefs to change.

After reading *Real Magic*, I wrote down a list of affirmations, and put them in my drawer by my make-up. When I pulled out my make-up, I pulled out the affirmations. I added to the list as I thought of positive thoughts that I would like to include in my life. I warned my husband that I might be talking to myself in the bathroom, but not to worry. I took my list on business trips. Some of my affirmations were taken from Louise L. Hay's book *You can Heal Your Life*. I'll share a few from my list.

- **My needs and desires are always being met.**

- **I am willing to give up difficulty, and learn my lessons with ease.**
- **Divine Intelligence gives me all the ideas I can use.**
- **Everything I touch is a success.**
- **There is plenty for everyone, including me.**
- **I am blessed beyond my fondest dreams.**
- **There are plenty of customers for my services.**

What happened in my life once I started to recite affirmations? I started to believe in myself. I asked the Universe to reveal my life's purpose. Teachers showed up in the form of books and people in perfect order. One of my first teachers came in the form of an acquaintance from work, Arlene Chemers. It had been many years since I had talked to Arlene. A series of phone calls lead to her. When I told her why I had called, she shared her life's work. To our mutual amazement and delight, she explained that it was her unrealized soul work to offer support and encouragement through seminars to people like me who wanted to find and follow their heart's desire. My phone call prompted Arlene to develop a focus group. Up to that time, she had not acted on her own heart's desire. It was at that group session that I admitted to others that I was very much ready to make a change in my life. Sharing my desire with others was an important and freeing step for me. After the focus group, books and life experiences continued to appear in my life until my answer came. As I mentioned earlier, this book you are reading is the result. I hope to continue with subsequent workshops, seminars and motivational speaking.

With these experiences I started to believe what Deepak Chopra wrote in his book, *Seven Spiritual Laws of Success*. In law number seven on Dharma, Dr. Chopra teaches that everyone has a purpose, something they do better than anyone else in the world. Now I'm writing down my experiences and self-publishing this book because I know that through the gracious support of the Creator, this book will find it's way to you. Writing this book has contributed to my healing, and I hope that your healing will start or continue as you read it.

After we find love for ourselves through affirmations, we need to show our newfound love by nurturing ourselves. Our relationship with ourselves is extended to those around us. If we don't know how to treat ourselves with heartfelt love and kindness, we will be unable to treat others with heartfelt love and kindness. If we do not treat ourselves with honor and respect, others will not treat us with honor and respect.

Many of us are not accustomed to nurturing ourselves. Much of our lives we've been nurturing those around us. We worry that doing it for ourselves will make us self-centered. Sometimes we may feel guilt about taking care of ourselves, when in reality it is truly the best gift we can give to those around us and ourselves.

Give yourself, something special, everyday. That was the advice I received from a spiritual individual after I told her that I had been giving a lot and was ready to start receiving. To me, she was a human angel.

We can give ourselves time. Julia Cameron suggests in her book, *The Artist's Way,* that we take ourselves on an artist's date once a week. Julia suggests we plan ahead to insure we have the time available to treat our artist within and ourselves. She also suggests we endeavor to avoid the temptation to bring along a third individual.

In addition to giving gifts to ourselves or taking time for a date. Here are more ideas for self-nurturing: soak your feet, soak yourself in a bath of aromatic oils, go to a movie, rent a movie you've always wanted to see, put on a favorite CD and dance around the living room, go for a walk and notice mother nature, go for coffee with a good book, eat your favorite food. My favorite? Prepare gelatin and drink it before it sets up.

Find what works for you and do it on a regular basis. You deserve it!

As we discover self-love we need to be aware of the powerful tool of our imagination. Add some feelings to that imagination, and it becomes even more powerful. Many times we review our feelings of anger and hurt over and over in our minds to justify their validity, and our right to feel them. And in the same way that positive thoughts can change our lives, so can the negative thoughts.

At a family session during treatment at The Recovery Center, the counselor brought out a "feelings chart"; a sheet of paper covered with facial expressions drawn into round circles. This sheet was created to help individuals like us to identify our feelings. Many of us had never identified our own feelings; we were so caught up in the feelings of those around us. We had become so entangled in our loved ones' lives that we abandoned our own feelings to nurture and help those we loved with their feelings.

One day I was experiencing extreme emotional feelings. I told my friend, Queen, that I worried I would break into tears at any moment. She reminded me that our feelings are our indication that we are really alive. She pulled an imaginary blanket close to her body and tucked her head inside while she shared how she liked to experience and feel her emotions. To Queen, emotion-filled days present an opportunity to celebrate life! A simple change in perception can bring with it the chance to find pleasure in all of our life experiences.

The "feelings chart" I shared earlier may seem funny or cute, but for me, it had a valid use. If we don't have a "feelings chart" to help with feelings or emotions, we can ask our Higher Power for help. We might choose to dissolve our fear-based emotions rather than celebrate the feeling of them.

We can become aware of the two energies in the world: love and fear, to help us on our path to discover self-love. Every emotion that we have is the result of one of these two energies.

We can learn to break down our fear-based emotions by simply identifying what fear caused the emotion. Fear is more tangible than our emotions, which makes it easier for us to distinguish whether or not it has merit. To transmute my fears, I think of my fear in its worst conceivable scenario, then recognize that even the worst possibility wouldn't be that bad.

We can transmute our fears by looking at fear without judgement. We can remember that there is nothing in this Universe to fear. In our perfect Universe, there is no right or wrong way to live. We can find meaningful purpose in all of our experiences. Since we tend to draw what we put our emotional energy into, it would be advantageous for us to dissolve our fears. I have an example of how power fearful energy can be.

Our miniature schnauzer, Sebastian got into some burrs and had a couple tangled in the fur on his underbelly. We didn't realize the burrs were there until they had caused him some irritation. My husband and I had to hold him down to cut the burrs out. He was nervous about us touching him in the tender area and cried out when we tried to get him to hold still. We finally got him on his back; he was shaking in fear as we found the burrs to cut them off. His fear was evident to our cat, Miracle, and she jumped onto the couch and started to bite him. Sebastian was drawing the pain that he feared.

Another emotion to be conscious of is Envy. Until we discover true self-love we may be tempted to practice envy. If we do, we are sending the message that what we have is inadequate. We are indicating that our Creator has given something to someone else that should have been ours. We are not trusting in the gracious gifts given to us by our Creator that are uniquely ours, and of value to all of creation. When we practice envy, we put a limit on our own possibilities and probabilities. Each of us is a unique individual with possibilities that are limitless and solely ours. Why would we ever want to abandon all of our experiences to take the opportunity of another? Instead, why not celebrate our differences, and know that our opportunities are solely ours, as are the opportunities of those around us?

# Chapter 9

## The Power of Manifestation

*We <u>are</u> capable of manifesting our desires, and thankfully our Higher Power knows what is best for us in our life.*

Recently, I left my former employer after twenty-two years to pursue a completely different career. Before I discovered the process I've shared with you throughout this book I would have been filled with fear. Now I can trust my Higher Power to guide me with each step I take. I do not know which path I will take until it is before me, and I follow that lead with acceptance that it is the will of the Universe. I will affirm that I desire success, but I will be careful not to define how

I think success will come to pass. When we define how, we take away the millions of possibilities the Universe has to offer us. When we define how, we limit ourselves.

I am a firm believer is manifestation. Once I started to ask the Universe for my life's purpose and believed that I would receive an answer, my life experiences became one miracle after another. All who know me are amazed at the changes that have occurred in my life in a little over a year and a half. I have never been happier. I thank my Creator daily for the opportunity to feel this much joy. As I wrote earlier, before I could believe and receive, I had to change my long held beliefs of limitation and unworthiness. You too can receive the bountiful gifts from the Universe.

We can learn to trust and accept the gracious gifts of the Universe with a fuller understanding of our Higher Power.

We <u>are</u> capable of manifesting our desires, and thankfully our Higher Power knows what is best for us in our life. Our Higher Power acts as a patient parent allowing us to experience pain and discomfort for growth.

We've identified some reasons why we have not trusted our Higher Power, and accepted the gracious gifts available:

**1. We could be harboring some disabling beliefs regarding the availability of our Higher Power.**

**2. We didn't think we were worthy to go before our Higher Power with a request.**

**3. We think we are being punished.**

**4. Our prayers were being answered, but in a way that was unrecognizable to us.**

After I worked through the beliefs that were keeping me from the unconditional love of my Higher Power, I found that I could ask for and receive immediate answers. This benefit was shown a few years ago when I received an immediate answer to a request.

I was lying in my bed reading the book, *We Don't Die* by Joel Martin and Patricia Romanowski. The book is about the gifts of medium George Anderson. George has the ability to communicate with individuals who have died. Many bereaved relatives contact George when they need reassurance that their deceased loved one does experience life after death. I came to a part in the book that left me feeling uneasy.

George had received a call from a woman. The woman had finally started to find peace in her life after many years of struggle, only to discover that she had cancer. She wanted George to tell her that she would continue to live physically, but George reminded her that she already knew what was inevitable.

After reading this story, I started to feel fear regarding my own death. I put the book down, closed my eyes and asked that the fear be taken from me.

Soon after, a scene came into my mind. In it, I was coming in the back door of my childhood home in Lava Hot Springs, Idaho. I saw my mother and my dog, both deceased, standing by the kitchen sink. They looked at me, but neither moved toward me. There was a feeling of peace as we looked at one another. I was carrying a large heavy suitcase. I put it down just inside the door and felt immense relief when I did. The kitchen was bathed in a warm amber hue that sent feelings of acceptance and peace through my being.

The vision gave me feelings of relief, wellbeing and comfort. I felt the overwhelming delight of coming home. I believe I was getting a taste of the feeling we get when we die. The feeling was so pleasant that I brought the experience back to my mind many times throughout the following week. Today as I write about the revelation, my body tingles with confirmation of its truth. I don't fear death any longer.

It seems as if one day I was asking for a personal relationship with my Higher Power, and before I knew it I was joking with and celebrating that which is my Higher Power!

When we ask for a personal relationship and it becomes so, we are manifesting. Manifestation is the ability to ask for our desires, and have them come to pass. Some people call this technique prayer. Practicing manifestation might seem as though it is contrary to the concept of "a plan" I shared earlier. We might say, "if there is "a plan" then why manifest? Why not just kick back and let life happen?" In "a plan" concept, we are participants of a much larger plan where all things work together for the benefit of all. There might be several paths we can take, but ultimately we end up as one with creation. For an example, we might decide to go to the store. That decision brings with it many choices: we might crawl, we might walk, we might ride our bike or we might drive our car. Any of these choices will get us to the store. Some of our choices might take longer, and some might be more difficult. We might want to manifest taking the easy route to the store from now on.

Some of us may have difficulty accepting the gift of manifestation because we have set beliefs on how we think life should be lived. We might still be judging experiences as good or bad. Some of our beliefs might be: if it's easy it's not worth it; going without is saintly; humility will lead us to heaven; money is evil and money is dirty. If we hold any of these beliefs—-and since our thoughts (beliefs) create our experience, we are in a cycle of taking the hardest path to the store. We believe that going to the store has to be difficult, or it's not worth the trip, so our thought (it has to be difficult) creates our experience (we crawl to the store). Again, it's our judgement based on beliefs that prevents us from finding peace, joy and happiness. We hang onto an old belief even if it's to our detriment. Some of us think we are unworthy and deserve to be punished, so we continue allowing ourselves to take the more difficult way. Discomfort does come with lessons, but wouldn't it be to our advantage to learn the lesson with less difficulty, then use the excess energy for experiences that make a contribution to humanity? We are all going to the same place (the store), so let's manifest taking a limo!

A great book came along at the perfect time in my life to help me manifest my life's purpose (the book you are reading). It's called, *Creating Money, Keys to*

*Abundance*, by Sanaya Roman and Duane Packer. Two entities, Orin and DaBen channel the contents of the book. They dedicate the book with the following statement:

> *To the spirit of abundance that is in each of you. May you recognize your greatness, discover your path, and make the contribution you came to make.*

Their statement takes our seemingly selfish request to manifest abundance, and transforms it into a much grander request: a request to discover our life's purpose! Our request to manifest abundance becomes a plea to help us find and fulfill our gift to humanity. A gift that only we can offer through our unique qualities.

I have always had a desire to manifest a contribution to humanity. During a psychic reading by Salt Lake City area psychic, Betty Finnas, I asked if she could see my life's work in the cards or on my palms. She told me that my purpose in this life was to experience joy. I was disappointed. For me to experience joy seemed like a rather selfish life purpose. I figured that meant that I wouldn't be making any sort of contribution to humanity. You can probably already see what I couldn't, but I was too close to the situation to see it until August 1998 when the idea for this book and subsequent seminars/workshops came to me. Ralfee Finn of, 7 Avenida Vista Grande, Suite B7-211, Santa Fe, NM Fe 87505-9199 wrote the horoscope reading I read in our local event newspaper, the

*Catalyst.* Ralfee specializes in Transformational Astrology. Her reading read:

> *The energy of the eclipses is catalyzing your desire to be of service. Excellent. Just keep in mind: be authentic in your choices. Remember, service isn't about sacrifice. It's about increasing your joy.*

Reading it again brings tears to my eyes. See how everything starts to work together in meaningful coincidences. It proves that there is a force much larger than we, at work in our lives.

Asking to manifest our desires is not being selfish. Forget all of the myths about money—-it is not evil. It is an external source. Despite the fact that it can't be our pathway to discover peace, it's not evil.

For me, manifesting money wouldn't work until I learned that I was the one keeping it from me. I had believed in limitation (there is only so much), and judgement (I had to be good before I could get some). To get past these two roadblocks, I had to change my beliefs about money. I discovered that I avoided using the word money in my affirmations. It was probably because I had strong feelings of being unworthy.

Even with the encouraging statement listed earlier, from the book *Creating Money, Keys to Abundance*, many of us still continue to have judgement about manifesting. We might not feel we are worthy to go before God and ask for our needs and desires. We might feel uncomfortable with the word manifesting. Some of us might feel more comfortable with the word prayer.

The term manifesting might make us feel as though we are taking over God's creating power. Many of us might view becoming creators as sacrilegious, when, in fact, we are creating our experiences with every thought that pops into our mind. Many of us have created unpleasant experiences unknowingly with our negative thoughts and words. We need to realize the things that work in our lives are a result of the good will and other positive qualities we have. A penetrating self-assessment will reveal we have indeed come a long way and have much to be proud of. We could use our creating power to our benefit if we started to become more aware of our thoughts. Becoming aware is a very simple way to change our lives. The Creator entrusted us with the power to create. We should use it wisely.

Since creating resides in our thoughts, we can manifest anything we can imagine. If we have asked for something, and we thought we believed, but we didn't get what we asked for, I'll review the four possible reasons why: 1) we did get it, but in a form that was not recognizable to us, 2) inside, we had a stronger contrary belief that negated our request, 3) it will happen, but later in our life, 4) our request is not beneficial to our higher purpose ("the plan" for our lives). I don't view humanity as spoiled children off creating their hearts desire no matter what the consequences. I see humanity in contact with its Creator working through a much larger picture that will one day come together, and show us a much grander plan than we could ever imagine.

We can use our imagination to manifest for our benefit. It brought us to this point, perceived skeletons and all. It's important that we trust that we are one with our Creator. We have the power to use our imagination to manifest goodness in our lives right now. There is no such thing as being worthy or unworthy.

As I mentioned earlier, *Creating Money, Keys to Abundance,* gave me the information I needed to make my book a reality. In their book, entities Orin and Daben communicate through authors Sanaya Roman and Duane Packer that we can help make our prayers a reality by imagining the feelings we expect to get with our answer. They suggest that we borrow a feeling from a past experience, and use our imagination to feel it while we manifest/pray. I needed money and time to write and self-publish this book. The feeling I needed was one of accomplishment. I borrowed the way I feel when I get compensated for services rendered. I imagined that feeling of accomplishment while I wrote imaginary checks for publishing costs from an account that had an abundance of money. I used the same feeling of accomplishment as I imagined the book completed and in the bookstore. Something remarkable happened. In late October 1998, my supervisor told my four fellow co-workers and me that management had decided to reduce our department in Salt Lake City by one coordinator. He offered an enhanced severance package to the employee willing to leave. The severance offer was based on the number of years of employment—-the more years, the larger the offer. Making the decision to leave after twenty-two years was frightening. But the offer looked like an answer to my prayers. If I left, I would have the time I needed to complete my book and concentrate on my business while drawing an income. If I decided to stay, my decision would be fear-based, founded on the belief that the company was more capable of supporting my needs than the Universe. If I stayed, I would be sending a powerful message to the Universe that I didn't trust its capability to give graciously. This opportunity was an amazing reminder of the unlimited possibilities and probabilities of the Universe. I would have never imagined (while I manifested using feelings of accomplishment) that such an offer would come my way. When I asked for help, I imagined the resources coming available to complete the book. I allowed the Universe to decide how that would happen. I was surprised and delighted with the resulting offer. The offer helped me to know that this book is an important step to take at this time in my life.

Sometimes we manifest discomfort in our lives by bringing up our negative feelings, and playing them over and over again. Since feelings and imagination are a powerful combination, this practice can cause devastating results. I used to dwell on the negative aspects of my husband's drinking. I could see nothing, but negative. Now that I know how powerful my thoughts are I try to be aware of them, and keep them positive.

Try changing negative to positive. It will change your life!

Your answer to manifestation/prayer might come in a form that seems contrary to the request. As an example of this, my daughter prayed for a divine relationship. She was surprised when her husband asked for a divorce. The breakup was devastating at first, but before long she realized that the union wasn't the right one for her. She didn't get the answer she expected, but it was the right answer for her.

When my daughter sent out her manifestation, she did not tell the Universe how she thought her prayer should be answered. When we manifest in this way we allow the Universe to take us down the most advantageous path for everyone involved.

We've talked about the gracious gift of an intimate relationship with our Higher Power. We've reviewed that our Higher Power is desirous to aid us through manifestation. Now it is time to give thanks. If positive thoughts are powerful, imagine how much more powerful expressing gratitude is. The great part is, it's easy, and we can give thanks to our Creator at anytime. Expressing gratitude is extremely healing. I have a grand teacher—-an entity called P'Taah. I've studied P'Taah's healing teachings through channel Jani King, in his first book, *An Act of Faith*, then in his second book, *Transformation of the Species* and now with tapes and sessions.

P'Taah's teachings are very positive and life changing. They are full of the good news that the Universe is one, creation is in the process of creating, and each of us is an integral part of that whole.

P'Taah's latest teaching to me was on gratitude. He suggests that we sing our thankfulness every morning while showering, he says that the water is crystalline and very magnifying.

When I wake up depressed or unhappy, I start my day thanking creation for the goodness that surrounds me. I thank my Creator for my life, my family, my animals, my health, my challenges, my lessons, the beauty of Mother Nature, my ability to support my family and my beautiful home, and the means to pay for it. I like to acknowledge the warm water pouring over my body, and thank it, for the way it makes me feel. I hope I've prompted you to think about all of the things you are thankful for, and to remember to express gratitude for them.

# Chapter 10

## Universal Truths That Can Affect Your Life

*If the majority believes a certain way, we tend to question our own way of thinking.*

It is possible to experience the common belief held by the majority, but not necessarily by us. We can be affected by the ideas and fears of the majority without even being aware of it. The common belief may be contrary to what we think we believe, but it's what we continue to hear from the individuals around us.

If the majority believes a certain way, we tend to question our own way of thinking. A group of individuals may react in a way that an individual would never consider acting on their own. The riot following the Rodney King trial in Los Angeles is a perfect example of the pervasive influence of a common belief. We call it, gang mentality.

The common belief was shown to me during my career. I have caught myself thinking like the majority. I have been a proponent of gender equality. I've held the belief that inequitable gender treatment is still prevalent. My life experiences have been manifested according to that belief many times. I continued to draw inequitable experiences. Despite this belief, I have found myself at times entertaining the idea that the male needs to get paid more because he is the head of a household. It didn't make sense that I created that thought, because at the time I too was the head of a household. These ideas came from somewhere outside of me. Did I get the idea from pervasive energy around me, or did I hear it? Either way the common belief is powerful.

To combat the common belief, and my belief of gender inequality, I conducted an experiment. I started to say to myself that I was paid equitably according to the contribution that I made to the company. Within a month I received a promotion which helped to make that affirmation so. Our thoughts do create our experiences.

Another universal truth we can't escape is that each one of us is a part of creation. Even if we choose to take a difficult path, our loving Creator will "save" us and bring us into our position within the whole of creation. There is a grand plan orchestrated by our Higher

Power, and our "mistakes" are merely growing experiences to prepare us to take our place within the grand plan. As a part of creation, all things work together, our geographic location, our parents and the time period of our birth. They are all pieces in an overall scheme. Everyone we come in contact with is also a player in the same drama, and they too are learning the life lessons that they need to experience in this life. It is a difficult concept to accept using our physical brains. We might wonder how everything can be working together for the good of the whole.

An example of the whole of creation would be the way our body functions. Our body is made up of millions of cells working together to give us life. In the same way, the Universe is one creation with us playing our role as "universal cell" to give life to creation.

As a part of the whole of creation, the lessons we need to learn before we can take our place within it are happening daily. The individuals needed to help us learn the lessons are being drawn into our lives. If we choose not to learn the lessons, events will continue to come into our life until we learn what is needed. In the beginning, our life lessons may be fairly easy to learn, but as we resist taking responsibility by pushing the blame out to those around us, the lessons continue to come, growing in intensity

As you've read so far, I rebelled against learning my life lessons and prolonged my growing experience. It's not necessary to live a painful existence for many years of our lives. We can ask our Higher Power right now, for the ability to learn our life lessons with less difficulty.

There is also the universal truth we see as meaningful coincidences (synchronicity). They are happening in our lives all of the time. The events and people in my life have worked together with synchronicity to bring me to where I am right now. We can really see the synchronicity when we believe that all things work together for the benefit of all. Some of us fail to notice the meaningful coincidences because we haven't believed in "a plan". We've experienced coincidences, but have thought of them as a fluke. Noticing meaningful coincidences can be an exciting adventure. Each one is a piece of a puzzle coming together to make a picture full of meaning.

I have a fun example of synchronicity. I missed the birthday of my good friend, Chris. To make up for it I wanted to get her something special. I contacted my friend Carol Wheat and asked her if she had her handmade earrings with her. She told me, "no," but that she would bring them on Thursday. She approached me a day earlier, on Wednesday and said that she had the earrings that day. I had a particular dress of Chris' in mind, but worried that I wouldn't remember the unique colors. I walked by her and noticed that she had the dress on that day! Later when I reached into Carol's earring box, the first pair I pulled out was made of the exact colors I needed, and it was not a typical color combination. I told Carol that I wanted those colors, but that I didn't want that particular pair. She reached in and pulled out a second pair, and I said, "perfect!" I gave the earrings to Chris, and she loved them. She said that when she put the dress on that morning she thought to herself that she needed a pair of earrings to go with it. It was as if the earrings had been made especially for her, and knowing the spiritual nature of Carol, they probably were. That's synchronicity! Carol's earrings are not only beautiful, but she charges each pair with spirit fed positive energy.

It's fun to start to notice the events in our lives. We can ask our Higher Power where they are leading. We can thank the Universe for the adventure they offer.

So far in the book, I've told many stories to help you to open your mind to the availability of peace, joy and happiness in your life. In the same way that the Universe needs all of us to be whole, we need to incorporate the mind, body and spirit to make us whole. The following section includes ideas to bring together, mind, body and spirit.

# Chapter 11

## Mind, Body and Spirit

*Communion with our Higher Power is available, and it doesn't cost a penny. All we need to do is believe.*

Being whole by incorporating our mind, body and spirit is an important part of being human. In the Western part of the world, we traditionally haven't been taught the connection of the three. The ancient cultures, on the other hand, have believed in the connection for centuries. As medical costs sky-rocket, alternative practices have started to become an option in our health care. Many of the alternative practices are preventative measures to help keep our mind, body and spirit healthy.

The spiritual teacher Shakti Gawain in her audiocassette, *Four Levels of Healing*, believes that surface affirmations will not give us the level of healing we need for our physical, mental, emotional and spiritual health. In her audiocassette, she takes the listener on a path of discovery with exercises to discover the buried beliefs and rules we have created for ourselves through our lives. After each exercise, Shakti takes the listener into meditation to implement the new beliefs and rules. I recommend Shakti's, audiocassette, and her many inspired books.

Many teachers believe that affirmations are a good place to start. Affirmations are simple to implement, and if they are contrary to our core beliefs, our true beliefs will start to show themselves. At our core, we tend to have a problem saying one thing and believing another. When we start a regimen of affirmations, uncomfortable occurrences can start to happen in our lives. We are clearing out the old to make room for the new.

The unseen part of us knows what needs to be purged. It is available to help us as we walk down the path to healing and recovery.

All of the spiritual teachers today suggest meditation as a way to get in touch with our Higher Self or Spirit. Through meditation, communication with unseen beings is possible. Deepak Chopra suggests that we meditate two times for thirty minutes each day. As with all spiritual teachings, each of us should listen to the prompting of our Higher Power to select which form is best for us.

Meditation and prayer may be seen by some as one in the same. During meditation, however, the mind is cleared of all thoughts. Prayer, on the other hand, is a communion with our Higher Power. Use prayer to commune and meditation to listen for the guidance from our Higher Power.

I find that when I am busy doing a task that does not require conscious thought, I receive inspirational prompting from spirit. I experience a wonderful time of clarity while I bathe or shower and shortly after. I've taken a pad and pen into the bathroom with me, so that I won't miss a thing. Communion with our Higher Power is available, and it doesn't cost a penny. All we need to do is believe.

Spirit needs mind to commune with.

Blending our mind into the union of mind, body and spirit might seem like something we've already done. But our culture is immersed in the belief of individuality. While each of us needs to celebrate our uniqueness, we also need to celebrate our place as a part of creation.

In the same way we separate from creation, the mind separates from the body and spirit. This view is reflected in our western medicine. Despite what we have learned about our physical health, it takes mind, body and spirit working together for complete health. When was the last time our mind talked to our body? Actually talked to the cells, visualized healthy kidneys, asked the liver how it is doing, reminded the stomach of its important work. Talking to our body might sound silly, but the messages our body is hearing from our culture right now are mortality and deterioration. Read Dr. Deepak Chopra's book *Ageless Body Timeless Mind.* Start to bring the mind, body and spirit together with some inner body communication. No telephone needed.

Louise Hay, in her book, *You Can Heal Your Life*, believes that all disease occurs when we are in a condition of unforgiveness. As with any experience, disease is in our life to teach us something. If Louise is correct in her teaching, think how easily we could start to improve our health. Simply by discovering where we need to find forgiveness in our lives. Many of us might need hours of time alone to discover where we are harboring unforgiveness. In the same way that we bury disabling beliefs, we bury resentment.

Louise was inspired to create a listing of various diseases. She included in her list the reason for the ailment and an affirmation to repeat to facilitate a change in our belief. Louise suggests if her cause doesn't feel right, to go within and consult our Higher Power for the correct answer. Louise proved her theory by dissolving cancer in her own body.

Hatha Yoga can help maintain a body that is not only healthy, but is a joy to inhabit. I have been practicing Hatha Yoga for several years now. I'm still a novice, but that doesn't stop me. Hatha Yoga can be a nice alternative to traditional exercise. The stretching of Hatha Yoga feels wonderful.

I noticed my dog stretching into the yoga positions of lower dog stretch and upper dog stretch. I decided it would be wise, to do a few dog stretches five mornings a week. Although my routine doesn't compare to my dog's routine of practicing upper and lower dog stretch almost every time he gets up, it's a start.

Acupressure is another alternative health care solution we can do at home. It works off the same principles as acupuncture, except instead of needles our fingertips are used. Acupressure is an ancient Chinese technique. The fingertips are used to gently press specific points for specific ailments in the body. Acupressure is a way to do self-treatment. If used correctly, Acupressure will help the body release tension and promote blood circulation, which will aid in the body's natural ability to maintain health.

I practice Acupressure techniques each morning to relieve symptoms of PMS. I told my medical doctor that I had found relief for my PMS without using prescription drugs or surgery. Instead of being glad for me, my physician was suspicious and fearful that I was causing harm to my body. Western medicine techniques are often fear-based.

Sometimes, western medical attention is a necessity. I suggest you add to your medical routine the trust in your body's ability to recover.

Our body can aid in our continued good health. Many of us in the West haven't been taught this valuable belief. We've separated the mind from the body, thereby sending a powerful message to our body that we don't have faith in its abilities.

We can listen to our body for signals. Our body will give us a signal when we are receiving important spiritual information. My signal is chills that run up and down my body. For a friend of mine, it's prickles on the back of her neck. You too can get in touch with your signal.

We can further open our mind to the workings of the spiritual by becoming aware of our surroundings, and how we can use them to our benefit.

# Chapter 12

## Our Surroundings

*When you "put your house in order," it is like discovering a whole army of helpers you never realized was at your disposal.*

*Karen Kingston*
*Creating Sacred Space With Feng Shui*

The teachers of the ancient Chinese principle of Feng Shui, meaning "wind and water", believe that we can create harmony with nature by using balanced placement of the physical items around us. Karen Kingston writes in her book, *Creating Sacred Space With Feng Shui*:

> *When you "put your house in order," it is like discovering a whole army of helpers you never realized was at your disposal.*

Karen dedicates an entire chapter to clearing clutter. She believes that energy can become stagnant, and that clearing out the clutter can get it moving again. She indicates that clearing clutter is a way to help us get unstuck.

There is logic in the teaching of Feng Shui. In using Feng Shui, one would never place their desk in a position with their back to the opening. I know that when I'm doing business, I get a much better impression of a person seated behind a desk who is facing the opening to their office/cubicle. Not only do I get a better impression, the occupant feels more important. In addition, when the desk faces the opening, a visitor will not startle the occupant.

We might not have any input on the space we occupy at work, but we can incorporate some Feng Shui at home. Clearing clutter is a simple way to energize us. We'll find that army of helpers Karen mentions!

We can see the benefits of Feng Shui even if we don't believe in the teaching. We will feel better when we clean out our drawers and closets. It does feel good when everything is organized and in its place.

If we desire to purchase something new, we can make space for it by clearing out something we don't need or use anymore. Donate all of those items still in good condition.

In the same way that Feng Shui suggests that there is unseen energy being effected by our inanimate objects, there are living things effecting our surroundings.

Plants know who we are. When we talk to them, they talk back—-not verbally, but with peaceful energy.

My husband cares for the plants in our home. All of our plants are healthy with thick green leaves. They seem to reel with delight after my husband waters them, then stirs their leaves with his large hands. Our plants give off an aura of extreme fondness toward my husband.

In the book *How to See and Read the Aura*, author Ted Andrews suggests that hugging trees is very therapeutic. This may be something we choose to do in the privacy of our own yard, or in the quiet stillness of a forest.

# Chapter 13

## Simple Truths

*Internal health and wellbeing will effect*
*and change our external circumstances*
*so completely that it seems miraculous.*

Throughout the book it was my intent to share how I overcame the following ten revelations that have taken years to discover and grasp. In conclusion, I'll review each one.

**1. I was contributing to the unhealthy behavior.**

This one is pretty obvious if you read the whole book. Is it true for you as well?

**2. I needed recovery and healing too.**

As you found out from my experience, it is never too late to start finding healing and recovery. The first step becoming aware and admitting to needing healing and recovery.

**3. My own beliefs have prevented me from experiencing joy.**

Our reality is based on our beliefs and some of them are no longer beneficial to our wellbeing. We can simply change our life by finding and defusing these disabling beliefs.

**4. If I do not feel love for myself, I cannot give love.**

This is one of the most important truths. We can start to find our self-love, once we uncover and change our disabling beliefs.

**5. I have the power to change the beliefs that no longer work for me.**

Once we understand where our disabling beliefs came from, and why they no longer work toward our wellbeing, we can replace them with positive truths.

**6. My thoughts create my experiences.**

We can start to notice our negative thoughts. We can change them into positive thoughts. We can sit back and watch those positive thoughts change our life in positive ways.

**7. I have total control of my thoughts.**

While the external is out of our control, our internal requires our special attention. When we go inside we will find all of our answers.

**8. I have no control over the actions of others.**

I hope I've helped you to understand the fruitlessness of trying to control external circumstances. External circumstances have many variables, and we have control over none of them. The alternative to external control is internal understanding and healing. Internal health and wellbeing will effect and change our external circumstances so completely that it seems miraculous.

**9. Everything works together for a purpose.**

With trust in our Higher Power, we can start to see our place in the overall universal plan where everything works together for good.

**10. The discomfort doesn't go away, but it lessens with changed perceptions and becomes an adventure.**

Our entire existence can positively change if we start to see each discomfort as a challenge and an adventure.

# Chapter 14

## My Belief

*This plan is bigger than our physical world, yet it can fit into our hearts. It is my prayer that you find peace, joy and happiness.*

I believe in a grand plan. This plan is bigger than our physical world, yet it can fit into our hearts. I believe that we can all find peace, joy and happiness. These three precious gifts are free, and available from our gracious Creator. It is our disabling beliefs that prevent us from receiving our birthright. We can change our beliefs to accept and receive them at any time.

The order of the Universe is based on what is so. That truth is very simple and unchanging. We have the power to choose our own way of seeing things. Each one of us individually has control over our own reality. To each of us, our perceived reality becomes truth, a creation. Although we have freedom to change our reality, we cannot change the Universal truth. Creation is very patient with her children, she allows them to go out to play, but she knows they will come right back to her. In the same way, we can set out to fly around the world, only to end up right back where we started.

Let's dance up the path of peace, joy and happiness. Let's allow the tears of peace to flow, and let's feel in our heart the overwhelming gifts of joy and happiness.

Gee, I learned a lot, I hope you did too.

# About the Author

After twenty-four years in the corporate environment, Brenda Ehrler was offered the opportunity to make the switch from corporate employee to small business owner. She started the publishing company***, Just Be Publishing, Inc***., to publish her non-fiction book written to aid in the healing and recovery of the friends and family members of the substance-addicted. It was Brenda's own healing and recovery from living with a substance abusing individual that led her to follow her heart's desire and reach out to others like her with books, tapes and motivational speaking. Brenda lives with her husband, their son and their kitten in Salt Lake City, Utah.

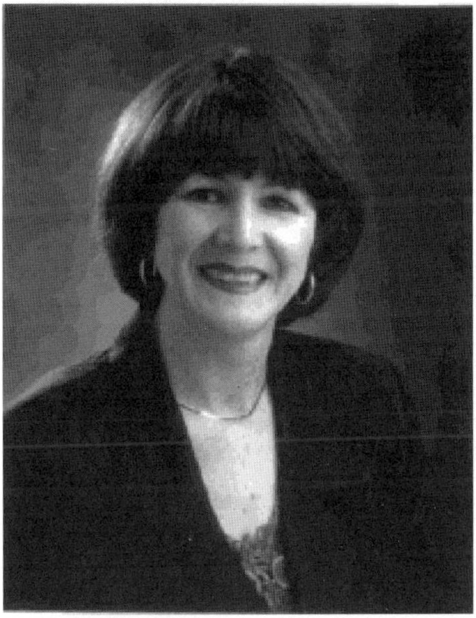

# RESOURCES

## BOOKS


Andrews, Ted. (1997). *How to See and Read the Aura.* St. Paul: Llewellyn Publications.

Cameron, Julia. (1992). *The Artist's Way: A Spiritual Path to Higher Creativity.* New York: G. P. Putnam's Sons.

Chopra, Deepak. (1994). *The Seven Spiritual Laws of Success.* San Rafael: Amber-Allen Publishing.

______. (1993). *Ageless Body, Timeless Mind: The Quantum Alternative To Growing Old.* New York: Harmony Books, a division of Crown Publishers, Inc.

Dyer, Wayne W. (1992). *Real Magic.* New York: Harper Paperbacks, a division of Harper Collins Publishers.

Friel, John, and Friel, Linda. (1988). *Adult Children: The Secrets of Dysfunctional Families.* Deerfield Beach: Health Communications, Inc.

Gach, Michael Reed. (1990). *Acupressure's Potent Points.* New York: Bantam Books.

Hay, Louise L. (1984). *You Can Heal Your Life.* Carson, CA: Hay House, Inc.

King, Jani. (1991). *An Act of Faith.* Perth, Australia: TRIAD Publishers Pty. Ltd.

______. (1991). *Transformation of the Species.* Perth, Australia: TRIAD Publishers Pty. Ltd.

Kingston, Karen. (1997). *Creating Sacred Space With Feng Shui.* New York: Broadway Books, a division of Bantam Doubleday Dell Publishing Group, Inc.

Martin, Joel, and Romanowski, Patricia. (1989). *We Don't Die.* New York: Berkley Publishing Group.

Maltz, Maxwell. (1960). *Psycho-cybernetics.* Englewood Cliffs: Prentice-Hall, Inc.

Nakken, Craig. (1988). *The Addictive Personality.* Center City: Hazelden Foundation.

Roman, Sanaya, and Packer, Duane. (1988). *Creating Money: Keys to Abundance.* Tiburon: H. J. Kramer, Inc.

Stone, Hal, and Sidra Stone. (1989). *Embracing Ourselves.* San Rafael: New World Library.

Wilde, Stuart. (1996). *Infinite Self.* Carlsbad: Hay House, Inc.

## PERIODICALS

Finn, Ralfee. (1998, August). "*The Aquarium Age.*" *Catalyst.*

## AUDIOCASSETTES

Gawain, Shakti. (1996). *Four Levels of Healing: A Guide to Balancing the Spiritual, Mental, Emotional and Physical Aspects of Life.* Mill Valley: Nataraj Publishing.